I See FAT PEOPLE!

Discovering Your 6th Sense...

of Eating!

By David Hrncir

DEDICATION

Thank you to my loving wife, Mary, and my wonderful children for your encouragement in everything 'Daddy' does. I love you!

CONTENTS

Acknowledgments   i

1   Fatroduction   1

2   The Disclaimer   4

3   Hooami   5

4   Is Fudge Eating Normal   9

5   Charging for Fat   11

6   Do These Genes Make Me Look Fat   15

7   $E=MEFAT^2$ 19

8   Back to the Fudger   29

9   I Dream of Eating   34

10 I'll Take a Side-of-Lucidity before the Meal   43

11 Too Fat or Not Too Fat, That is the Question   53

12 Couch Potato, Couch Potato, Who is the Couch   64
    Potato

13 Stop and Smell the Home Cooked Meal   76

        Appendix A. Lucid Dream   86

        Appendix B. What the Author Does   90

        Appendix C. Feed Me   100

ACKNOWLEDGMENTS

I would personally like to thank my body for all of the torture I put you through just to prove a point. I know that common sense should have just told me what was right. But regardless, you stayed with me. Thank you for being at my sides, my front, my back, my top, and my bottom. I hope that we can stay together and have many more happy years of life here on this wonderful planet!

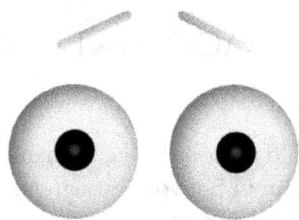

1. FATRODUCTION

I have an ugly secret...I see fat people! I know...what a way to begin a book right? No slow starts, no subtlety, just the plain truth. I see fat people. They are everywhere. Worse is, there seems to be more and more fat people. It's truly an "energy" epidemic. So what do we do? We read this book!

I have read about 10,000 books, online documents, etc. about eating. Alright, that may be a slight exaggeration. You name it, I've researched it...from the craziest diet, to the zaniest workout. And you know what I found? They all work. Yep, they all work. Now you are probably thinking, "Huh?" You read me correctly. All legitimate diets work. All legitimate exercise programs work. It's true. But...if that's the case, then why does it seem that everyone around me is getting fatter? People are getting fatter because exercise and diet programs work...while you do them, and most are unsustainable. Therefore, most people will not do them. And the people that do, usually fail because the programs require a tremendous amount of work and "above normal" program dedication to maintain their effects.

I'd be willing to bet you have not read a book like this one. I don't have 37 chapters on what your meal plan should be. I don't draw out complex exercise routines over 10 chapters that you must do for the rest of your life or you will fall back into what I call the "flump", the fat-slump. I simply share with you my amazing discoveries of enlightenment, nirvana, and true inner peace. Oh man, that is so not true; I laughed writing that. Nirvana and inner peace...probably not so much, but enlightenment is hopefully going to happen quite a bit.

This book will expound some ideas that may seem complex at first, but are very simple once comprehended. This book was engineered to be enlightening, educational, fun, and read in three to six hours. It makes no sense to give you complex stories about ideas that are easily explained in a shorter format. I think most people will agree with my short, to the point approach.

So, who needs this book? EVERYONE! No really, everyone. Some people are out there thinking, "Well I'm thin", or "I have a naturally fast metabolism." You may be thin. You may have a fast metabolism like I used to have, but you may know people who do not. You may have friends or family members that have tried every diet and exercise plan known to man, woman, and homo-sasquatches, all of which have ultimately failed. Also, what about the people who truly do not have time to exercise on a daily basis? Or want to? All of them need this book.

I promise you, this book is different. Again, I don't tell you how to exercise. I don't even define what a balanced meal is. This book is designed to attack "fat" from an energy point of view; that's why it's different...and that's why it will change the way you think about food and the process of eating. Just to warn you though, this book is not all about being serious, in case you haven't noticed that yet. Not all health information has to be mundane. I believe if you can maintain an inquisitive, humorous attitude while reading, you absorb information very easily.

Therefore, this book contains my feeble attempt at humor to keep your spirits high and to keep you from going into shock from information overload. I do not want you slipping off to sleep, so I'll try to keep the topics fun and chapter changes smooth. I really tried to keep this book short and to the point. So if it's too long, then you are a very slow reader...which may good...pace yourself!

And now I would like to present something that is amazing. It's incredible, astonishing, and breathtaking at times...

2. THE DISCLAIMER

That right folks, the DISCLAIMER! Because of ridiculous lawsuits brought about by people who think a book alone will change them into lean, mean, kings and queens, and that a book when rubbed on your thighs will melt away fat, I have to make the following statements. This book is in intended in no way, shape, or form to cure any illness or disease or give you any kind of weight loss results of any kind. Everything in this book is my opinion, and should be received as so. I do not offer any physical or nutritional plans. Even when I write the word "you" in the book, I am really talking about me in 3rd person, even though I really don't like when people do that. This book will not allow you to leap tall buildings. It will not give you winning lottery numbers. It won't even hold the door open. Ok, that's a lie. If you jam it in a door that is closing, most likely, it will hold the door open…unless it's an electronic version.

Disclaimerrrrrrrrrr…done!

3. HOOAMI

Some of you who read the chapter title probably thought, "Is this a type of sandwich...or yoga position?" "Who am I?" I asked myself that question because, truly, who am 'I' to write this book? Well there should be a picture of me somewhere in this book, but that's not what I mean. So many times we put our faith in someone based on who they say they are by listing out credentials or a pedigree as if that makes them an expert in how "my" body works. Sometimes we put all of our faith in a person because they have "PHD" behind their name. Sorry, my suffix only goes to "BBA". I had a professor with a PHD in college tell me, "David, don't take as fact what someone with a PHD tells you; research it yourself. Because you know what PHD stands for right? Piled Higher and Deeper!"

I am just a regular person, as opposed to an irregular person. I am not of noble birth. Even though I am in pretty darn good shape, I am not a fitness instructor with 10 videos on how to sculpt your body. I can cook, but I am also not a nutrition specialist with recipes that will change your life. I'm a

40+ year old, father of four who has seen and documented what works on me, and I'm here to share the answer to the fat phenomenon with you. I want you to understand that I'm not here to preach; I'm here to share, and have some fun along the way. In case you haven't noticed, I tend to be more on the "lighter" side of things. I think making things that are interesting fun is just…well, better. You know how you have the glass half empty or glass half full people? Well, I'm one of those "it's just a glass of water" people…a straight shooter. I mean, just look at the chapter names. Ok, maybe not the best example; the chapter names are a bit riddling, I'll admit. But that's just part of the fun.

This book does have some serious findings though; I mean, I would never take fat lightly. The title of the book, of course, is a play on words. It is meant to be funny, and literal, but not mean. One thing about me, I am not mean; just blunt. People do not like being fat, no matter what they say. I know…from experience!

So at this point, if you are thinking, "Well since this guy is not a doctor or fitness instructor, I better just quit reading." Then quit. No, don't quit. I wasn't being serious…come on, give me and yourself a break. I think people like you are ready for a book like this one and from someone who will give a lot of awesome information in laymen's terms and not scientific mumbo-jumbo. So let us begin initialization of our cerebral cortex neural activity to a level of perpetual information absorption. Just kidding; no really…turn on your brain.

One thing I want to point out is that I have done a ton of research on myself. That's how I was able to write this book. That's another process that makes this book different. I didn't go out and research a bunch of topics that someone else has already done and just regurgitate it here; I try not to regurgitate. Seriously though, I had to figure this out on my own because all of "their" stuff just didn't work. Or it would work for a period of time, but then I would be right back where I started. Most importantly, I wanted to figure out how to control my fat percentage without changing my diet. That was the kicker, and why it took me over two years to get to this point. Yes! I said that early in the book...I did not change my diet to solve the fat problem. I also did not increase my exercise. As a matter of fact, I decreased my exercise, but more on that later. So the content I present in this book, and some of it cutting edge if you ask me, is what worked for me and continues to work with no effort whatsoever. Why is that important? Because isn't that what we are all seeking...how to stay in our normal fat percentage range with very little effort? Also, my findings are important because I am the average "Joe"...well..."David." Plus, I am getting so tired of those ads on every other web page showing a man or a woman with ripped abs stating that this could be me in four short weeks...yeah right! I wanted to document what "really" works for the long term.

So now that you still don't know who I am, what is in the book? A lot; really, a lot. But you know what? Most of the concepts and ideas I present to you will later become common sense and every day thought. That is the cool part. To me, and I bet to you too, this book contains a lot of common sense about uncommon knowledge. We understand the five senses already. We hear the food being cooked, smell the aroma, see the wondrous dish, touch the food to our mouths, and taste the deliciousness! The "big butt" is that we seem to have forgotten the sixth sense of eating, and that is where our problems lie. More importantly, that's what this book will help you come to realize and ultimately control!

The book has some ideas that will hopefully be a "ding-ding-ding" in your brain. Most of the ideas I present in the book seem to be missing from the average person's consciousness. How do I know? I was one of them. The ideas and processes I present in the book describe how our lack of understanding in regards to energy consumption has created an obese society. But the great thing is, the processes for which I am referring are easy…to understand and perform. Again, I kept the chapters short because I like switching topics to keep you on your toes. I think you'll like it because each chapter leads into the next one; what a novel concept. So just when you think you won't get the answers…

Sorry, I really couldn't help myself. You will get the answers! And you're going to be shocked at how simple the answers are.

Ok, who's up for fudge?

4. IS FUDGE EATING NORMAL

I wanted to start this book by giving a quick eating scenario. How about we create a fictitious character named "Elmer Fudge"? We will refer back to this scenario throughout the book. Here's Elmer on an average day. Can you relate?

Elmer wakes up and for breakfast eats a bowl of fiber-rich cereal with 2% milk, drinks an 8 ounce glass of orange juice, and drinks one cup of coffee with creamer. Hmm....not bad. During the morning at work, for which Elmer is a software engineer, Elmer has a small bowl of peanuts and 4 ounces of an 8-ounce cola as a mid-morning snack. Elmer eats a deli style sandwich, small bag of chips, and drinks a sweet tea at lunch. For a mid-afternoon snack, Elmer eats one small candy bar and drinks the other 4 ounces of cola. For supper, Mr. Fudge eats two pieces of fried chicken, a small serving of mashed potatoes and gravy, some broccoli, 8 ounces of iced tea, and small piece of cheesecake.

Now you are probably thinking of a couple of things. First, of course, is why I was so smart as to *not* use a copyrighted name as my character. Second, as to why the scenario is described at this point in the book. And third, I wanted you to see a more "real" scenario. Ok, this is truly more of a healthy scenario, but still a real scenario. Does it read like a good scenario? Do you think it sounds healthy, unhealthy, or in the middle? Wrong. Just kidding. There is no correct answer, or is there?

Now let's do a breakdown of the above scenario into approximate calories since we know everything in the world revolves around calories. Let's say his breakfast was a good 400 calories, mid-morning snack at 300 calories, lunch at 700 calories, mid-afternoon snack at 300 calories, and a dinner at 800 calories. That's an approximate total of 2,500 calories for the day. Not too bad considering Mr. Fudge is 6 foot 2 inches and about 210 pounds. This will come into play later in the book. So our scenario is set.

You know what's awesome? The next nine chapters are going to have all of the basic information I want to share with you. The rest of the book, you can rip out and throw in the trash.

Please don't rip out the rest of the book and throw it in the trash…especially if you have not paid for the book yet or borrowed it from a friend.

Let's energize!!!!

5. CHARGING FOR FAT

I like this chapter…mainly because I wrote it. First, a little bit of scientific mumbo-jumbo. The term "calorie" is used widely because we can easily rate food by caloric intake. Now there are so many other food factors besides calories, but for our discussions here, we are going to use calories as our focal point. Remember, this book is written to solve the fat phenomenon from an energy point of view; so I will not list details about perceived health benefits from various types of food. I basically treat all food as equal in this book. The food's calories are my concern.

You can find this anywhere, but a calorie is just a measurement of heat energy needed to raise the temperature of a gram of water one degree Celsius; in human terms, the energy needed to move our booties on this wonderful planet. Ok, that's about as scientific as I am going to get. I do feel smarter now. One calorie is the equivalent to around 4.184 joules. Ok, now I feel really smart. Enough of the science stuff.

What does that mean…the definition of a calorie…and how it relates to my body? I don't know. Did you ever say that? "I don't know what calories in my body actually mean." I did; seriously. Someone would say, "You know that candy bar is 400 calories." I would reply, "Yep, and my truck is dirty." I didn't know what to say. Maybe "Thanks." Or maybe, "Good thing I ate it really fast so it didn't explode and kills us all!"

So then I realized something; I wasn't dumb, I just didn't have the experience. (Flashback: My mother once told me, when I was 18 and knew everything, that I really was ignorant of life and that age would bring me wisdom. My poor mother, hmm, hmm, hmm…she was right.) Now, once again, before some scientist comes along and spends a 1,000 hours and 500 algorithms as to why I'm incorrect…remember…this is what worked for me. And since I am just the average guy, I bet will work for you too. So take that scientists! I mean, we all know what calories are, kind of; we just don't know fully how they work in our body. Or, more importantly, how they are stored and used by our body.

Alright, prepare your brains…humans equate to rechargeable batteries. No really. Truthfully, every animal does. We need energy to live. All life needs energy. Without an energy source, life ends. So let's go back to what I just stated. Rechargeable batteries, hmm. For a battery to be useful to us for an electric purpose, it needs to be charged. Rechargeable batteries, like humans, have evolved over time. I like to think we, as humans, are stronger and overall better today than humans were in the past. The same goes for batteries. We now have batteries that last longer and can hold a charge longer. But the concept is still the same. When a rechargeable battery's energy is spent, it needs to be recharged. Same goes for a human. When a human's energy is spent, a human needs to be, well, recharged.

Like a battery, we have different types of chargers

that can be used, i.e. different foods to give us different types of energy. Batteries usually have speed chargers or trickle chargers. Speed chargers for batteries quickly charge the batteries, but the energy does not last long and usually shortens the battery's life. Trickle chargers for batteries charge slower, but give batteries better endurance and longer life. These characteristics are almost the exact same as how humans recharge.

Speed chargers, bad carbohydrates for example, give humans a quick boost, but does not last long. Trickle chargers, good fats for example, are digested longer and are fed to our bodies at a slower rate and are therefore used at a slower rate. There can be problems and dangers when recharging. When we overcharge, or speed charge, batteries often, they tend to last a lot shorter than normal. If we severely overcharge the batteries, they die...meaning they lose all of their charge and their ability to hold charge. Humans are no different. If we constantly overcharge ourselves (overeat), we will speed up the process that limits our life.

Humans have one distinct advantage over batteries. Know what it is? We are not bound by a certain physical size. We can expand and contract as needed. The problem is we tend to expand more often than contract. So if we are just like rechargeable batteries which only need recharging when the energy is low, and we should just contract back to where we were before recharging, then why do I see fat people? Answer: Because they are right in front of me? Well yes, but that's not what I meant. I see fat people because many of us have become addicted to speed chargers.

Stop for a minute and absorb what I just stated. We may blame our lives and our extracurricular activities, but many of us have made the horrible choice of using speed chargers too often instead of trickle chargers. And by speed chargers, I don't just mean fast food. I also mean eating a vast amount of calories at one sitting. Right now, sit back just for about a minute and think about how many times a week, or month, you use speed chargers versus trickle chargers. Back already? Hey, you just didn't keep reading without thinking about how many times you speed charge per week did you? Don't cheat. "We" are reading this book for a reason right? It's truly sad how many times we speed charge without even realizing it. We know that most rechargeable batteries are made from various types of metallurgy components. What about humans?

Microscope please.

6. DO THESE GENES MAKE ME LOOK FAT

I see fat people; mainly because I look in the mirror to get dressed every day. Well, not too much anymore. No, I mean I still look in the mirror, but...well I still get dressed...ok, you know what I mean. The fat part! But boy was that not the case before...well, before I awoke my 6th sense. I have an engineering mindset. If something does not work, I simply go online and buy a new one. Wait...no...that's wrong. I meant engineers find a means to an end through trial and error and usually try to fix the minor issues versus chunking the whole project.

Engineers typically find what works from understanding what does not work. To remember what works, engineers create formulas. So I decided to set my engineering mindset on humans and food and why we get fat. So why can't we just stuff ourselves with whatever amount of food we want? Why can't we just eat what we want and have our bodies just "know" what to do? Come on, it can't be that complex. Can it? Well the answer is an amazing "yes". It is that complex...our bodies that is.

Humans have evolved over who knows how many millennia to have to scavenge for food. Technically, we are hunters and gatherers. Meals may have taken us hours or even days to acquire in the distant past. That type of food availability forced our digestive system to evolve into a system for which we may not totally agree, at least not in our current state of evolution. The point I'm trying to make is that we, as hunters and gatherers, store food as fat when food is in abundance. The stored fat helps keep our "batteries" charged while we hunt and gather for more food. Of course now, we can drive to the grocery store in 10 minutes, or worse to the fast food restaurant in 1 minute. Not a whole lot of hunting or scavenging needed, but we still store fat as though we are still hunting and scavenging.

Here comes the complexity part. Humans have billions of codes and who knows how many of these billions of codes define how we store and use energy. So, needless to say, the codes that need to adapt to our "new speed charger mentality" just cannot adapt quick enough. And believe it or not, that is a good thing.

So let's touch on the fat shall we. Not literally, but theoretically. Here's the question: why do we even store fat? Too much storage makes me not fit into those jeans...stupid genes...or smart genes? Fat is our life force. It's contains nothing but pure nutrients and building blocks to help engineer and nourish our body's developing systems and energy needs. Take newborns for example. For the first year or so of life, all they need is mother's milk. What's in mother's milk? Mostly water and fats. What's in baby formula? Water, DHA, RHA, etc. What is that? Mostly water and fats. Without the fats, babies would not be able to develop into healthy toddlers.

So fats are used to engineer complex systems in our

bodies like neural development. How about polar bears? Boy that's a conversation starter! Why do polar bears, for the most part, eat only the fat from the animals they kill and leave the meat? Because they have evolved over time to know that the fat they eat will last them longer than the protein. Too, the time in between meals for polar bears can be extensive. The exact opposite is true for the giant cats on the Savannah. Since food is abundant, they do not need to store energy for too long; so they eat the protein instead for strength and leanness because they are required to hunt more often.

Humans are somewhere in the middle. We start out as polar bears needing primarily fat to grow, but once we get past a couple of years of age, we no longer need the high volume of fats, or really the high volume of calories, to sustain life. That stinks, especially when you love ice cream! As humans get older, we tend to be more like the cats where we eat more proteins than fat. So for older humans, is fat good, bad, healthy, unhealthy? Yes!

Now very quickly, depending on how fast you read, I'm going to put in a "disclaimer addendum". Some people…very few…but some people seem to have a genetic issue with fat storage being turned on in overdrive from conception. I truly believe this because I know some people who since the time they could take a step were fat no matter what they ate. The genes that control fat storage are just not mapped correctly and make it difficult to control the percentage of fat on their bodies no matter what they do. This book can still help those people regardless, but the uphill battle can be quite a bit more daunting for people who are genetically fat. So why did I state that? I'm "guess-timating" the people I am referring to are the 0.00001%. That is a very tiny percentage of our population. So don't try to cheat yourself by lumping yourself into that percentage when you are not genetically fat. Now, back to the 99.99999% of us; why do we get fat?

I have found the reason we store too much fat, and it's from...get this...eating! Yep. Can you believe that? Oh what? You want more than just that? Really? Just kidding. We get fat from not eating the wrong foods, but from <u>eating wrong</u>! Still want more? Man are you a glutton for punishment. I hoped so! And I'm going to give it to you...right now! Woo-hoo! I'm getting excited.

Formulation time!

7. E=MEFAT2

I know I shouldn't show favoritism, but this is my favorite chapter! Remember the old adage, "You are what you eat." I think what our parents and nutritional guides were trying to tell us is that if you eat junk food, then you are junk. That was probably the figurative sense anyway. I took that a little further...to calories. To me, "you are what you eat" means that if you consume too many calories, you become a giant battery! Wait! Before you slam the book closed and say, "This is when he tells us to count every calorie of every meal we eat during the day. Who has the time or the means to do that?" No. That is not what I am stating. Who has the time or the means to do that?

What I am stating is that we should count calories in generalities. Why count in generalities? Mainly because who knows the correct answer to how many calories we need per hour, per time of day, per day, and so on. Seriously, is someone going to tell you how many calories you need per day? Do they follow you everywhere you go? Do they know every single activity you do? If they do, I would seriously move and file a restraining order...that's creepy. If "they", and I love the ambiguous "they", don't know your body type, metabolism, exercise habits, etc., then how in the heck can they tell you or guide you by setting a caloric intake amount? Answer: "They" can't! There. I said it…well you know…stated it.

The best online formulas out there to get BMI, RMR, and more abbreviations than I care to list are not geared for every individual, and I would bet they are off +/- 15% at least. So while they are a great start, they are only part of the equation and should not be used solely. More on that to come as well. Keep reading; you're almost to it!

So is the Elmer Fudge eating scenario good or bad? If you said, "I don't know," then you are correct. We don't really know, do we? There are too many variables missing. What exercise did Elmer do and when? What is Mr. Fudge's caloric burn when he is at rest (RMR – resting metabolic rate)? Nope, we truly have no idea if that eating scenario is good or bad. So what do we do? How are we supposed to know how many calories we should be consuming per day?

The FDA states maybe 2,000 calories per day is fine for the average adult. A couple of nutrition web sites may state 2,500 calories per day is better for 'healthy, active' people. Then, you can go to 40 other places and find all kinds of variances. We could review a couple of them and find an average, but will "the average" be correct? Maybe. Some of the charts that show age, weight, height, etc. and give you a baseline can be a good start. To know for sure, you would need to perform a RMR test where you sit completely still for about 10 minutes and breathe into a machine that makes you sound like Darth Vader. RMR tests are not very expensive, and it's a one-time cost that could really benefit you in your life and for what I'm about to explain to you.

Once again, RMR stands for resting metabolic rate,

and this term is VERY important. I'll explain it more in a bit, but, basically, your RMR is the amount of calories you burn when you are totally idle. That is the number you need to know because your RMR is a major component of your eating guide...your baseline in other words. You have to know how many calories your body can burn when just sitting idle. If you do not have access to a facility that can perform a RMR test, you'll have to be a part-time engineer and do some trial and error before you get the right number. But do it because RMR is invaluable in regards to your 6th sense!

Seriously, we spend so much time on useless decisions such as deciding what type of TV we are going to buy next or learning how to program our DVR. We can at least spend a little time figuring out how our body uses energy. There are quite a few online RMR calculators if you initially want to go that route. Perform a couple of calculations from three or four and take the average. That will probably do for now. Once you go through the process I'm about to explain once or twice, you will be able to refine your RMR to a very precise approximation.

Let's say that Mr. Fudge has a moderately lean muscle build, exercises once or twice a week, and is 40 years old. That would mean Elmer burns about 2,000 calories per day when totally at rest (taken from RMR...not daily allowance). Not too shabby and is the norm for the average male around the age of 40. So if Elmer follows that eating scenario and does not exercise that day, what do you think happens? Yep, he has 500 calories that will not be used by his body within the day. That means the next time he consumes food or if his body stays in a long resting state, his body will store off the 500 calories as fat. Thank you genes!

Yep, that should have been a "wow" in your head.

This is what happens when you consume more calories per day than you can burn up. The reason that should be a "wow" is because the eating scenario seems like a pretty good one, but yet, Mr. Fudge fudged.

So why am I going on and on about Mr. Fudge? Well here's why. I'm pretty close to Mr. Fudge in caloric burn per day. I have about a 2,200 RMR per day. So here is what drove me crazy...why did I still gain weight/fat when I really controlled and, dreadfully, counted my calories? I am a pretty physically fit person. I was eating very close to my total calories per day based on my RMR, and my RMR was correct. The exercise I was performing should have burned up whatever excess I went over. So what was going on?

I was very upset at my body. Mostly, I was frustrated which is how most people feel when they just can't get the fat off by continuing what they think is a balanced diet. Why did I gain weight/fat if I ate good food and stayed close to my RMR per day? Being an engineer, I did my trial and error, and I figured it out. What I have discovered has completely changed the way I eat and has changed my life forever, and it is not just controlling the total amount of calories per day. Ready? You MUST control the amount of calories consumed per eating interval so as to not surpass your amount of calories burned between each eating interval based on your RMR per day!!!! KEEP READING! I just wanted to state that before you re-read the sentence I just wrote over and over. I was laughing as I wrote that because I know you're probably thinking, "Uh, did I miss the important part?"

Probably not the best way to present that at first, but in reviewing the sentence one more time, it is exactly what I meant to write. What do I mean? Simply put, you should try your hardest and teach yourself to NOT eat more calories than you can burn before the next time you eat. Ok, I guess that was a little easier to write, but didn't sound as scientific as the first sentence.

Now, I have to prove my point. Again this is what I found and what happens to me when I eat. I truly have no laboratory with people eating how I ask them to eat and then documenting all the results so that you can qualify the data. I have performed many experiments on myself. Why would I do that? Because I had to figure it out. Like I stated previously, getting fatter when I "thought" I shouldn't really made me upset.

Moreover, when I thought I should be losing weight and fat, I wasn't. Not losing weight and fat when I thought I should made me even more upset. Of course, I went a little overboard in my tests, but you got to do what you got to do. I did tests for which I knew I would get fatter…a lot fatter. Then did tests which should make me thinner. Then did multiple variances and crossovers to truly find out what was going on with my body. Yep, I pretty much felt like a lab rat.

One of the main discoveries I made is that if I consume a lot of calories, and then about two or three hours later exercise rigorously, I don't gain fat. I've done this over and over. I've eaten about 800 calories just hours before I swam a mile or more, and I did this for numerous consecutive days possibly changing my exercise routine, but still doing enough to burn close to 800 calories which is a lot of exercise…trust me. I never gained fat. I performed the daily measurements with calipers and tape measures over and over. I never gained fat or weight for that matter. On a side note, don't strictly use your weight as a guide for trying to be healthy. Again, who decides what your "healthy" weight should be? But measuring your weight daily in the morning after a little visit to the restroom right after you wake up is also a good baseline if you are concerned with weight and want to monitor your weight.

Now the contrary, when I ate in the same manner as I mentioned above, but did not exercise for more than a week and still consumed over 800 calories at one of my eating intervals a day, which put me around 3,000 calories for the total day, of course I gained fat. Here's the zinger on this test. When I went back and tried to eat normally (minus the 800 calories) and perform the rigorous exercise daily for the same number of days, to try to play catch-up basically, I discovered something pretty shocking when I performed my measurements...I was not back to the same size I was weeks before! HAAAA!!!

That finding hit me like a ton of greasy fries. What I found is that it is extremely hard to remove the fat once it's on me. After talking to quite a few people about burning their calories once they get fat, they agreed; it's tough. Once the fat is stored on my body, it is very difficult to get rid of it, especially if you have stored fat consecutively for long periods of time. Now I'm sure there are many factors as to why this happens, but I really do not care about that right now. The fat was stored, and it did not come off as expected. That is a fact. The entire purpose for the last few paragraphs is to assist in building my formula. Again, the engineer in me kicks-in.

I had to figure this out. Just as I outline how a system is going to be laid out and developed, I wanted to do the same thing for attacking this phenomenon. So what I have done, again this is just me, is I said that calories stored as fat are "super" calories...meaning they are stronger than the normal calories that are actively in your system waiting to feed your muscles. I am assuming the reason for this is that stored fat is concentrated energy, and that the body uses this concentrated energy more efficiently.

So how I altered my formula is when a calorie is stored as fat I multiply that calorie by 40% because that seems to be the additional perceived exertion needed to remove that fat. I'm sure some nerdy guy will come back later and document that it's actually 33.284% and prove me wrong, but he doesn't know how my body works like I do. Come on, perceived exertion is objectively subjective anyway.

Regardless, I'm just trying to show that to get the fat off, the amount of caloric reduction needed or the amount of additional exercise needed is increased by approximately 40%. This means if I do not exercise an additional 40%, I will not get that fat off. Of course, the type of exercise makes a huge difference; more on that in a later chapter. But the horrible fact that just bounced around like a crazy-ball in my head is that if I go back to my normal routine after gaining fat...I just keep the fat. I don't like that...not one little bit! So what did I do? I figured it out. Since I knew the processes that did NOT work, and I did not want to forget what "did" work, I did what engineers do; I created a formula.

Ok. Now before you even look at the formula, please do not fret about how strange it may appear or how you are going to memorize it. You do not really need to memorize the formula. How we apply our caloric values to the formula is much simpler. I created a formula just to have a scientific frame of reference for me. So, if you are not a formula person or if you are and I wrote this incorrectly, just skim this real quick and go to the next paragraph. So here it is....well on the next page.

Formula

(X ~ ((CCI:# - RMRFI:#) > 0 ? * 1.4)++) = TCSB

Legend

X – Random number of times a person consumes calories in a day.

CCI# – A specific Calorie Consumption Interval. (Eating, more importantly, eating anything with calories.)

RMRFI# – A specific Resting Metabolic Rate Fasting Interval. (Calories burned based on RMR between meals or between consumption of calories not associated with exercise.)

TCSB – Total Calories Stored/Burned. (Positive is calories stored as fat and negative is "stored fat calories" burned.)

> 0 ? * 1.4 – States if the previous calculated value is positive, then multiply by 40%.

++ – Add up all of the calculated values together.

I know…as my sister would tell me…what a geek. So here is how you read the formula. Take the calories you eat for a meal (CCI#1) and subtract the calories you burn for the time between this meal and the next meal (RMRFI#1). If the value for that difference is positive, add 40%. Do the same for every meal you eat (X being the variable of total meals per day) which will most likely have a different amount of calories for the meal and a different amount of time between the prior meal and the current meal; that's what the 'X' represents. Add all of the differences together to get the total (TCSB). If the total number is positive, fat was stored. If the total is negative, fat was utilized or "burned" to create energy and, therefore, was not stored.

Now remember, this formula is based on a day where you do not exercise. As you can see from the formula, I purposefully left off the subtraction of calories burned from exercise. The reason for this is because you may exercise at different times during the day. You would need to insert your subtraction of calories burned from exercise into the correct place in the formula. But again, this formula is geared for a day in which no exercise was performed. If you wanted to make it simple, you could just subtract your calories burned during exercise from the TCSB value. Then the former applies; positive, fat was stored, and negative, fat was not stored and most likely was burned…maybe depending on the type of exercise.

Ok wait! Please, before you have negative thoughts being upset because of the calorie counting and formulas, just keep reading because it makes more sense here in a minute. Remember I stated this was going to be an easy read? Trust me. It is. You'll see. You want a TCSB around 0 every day. That means you break even! Hooray! That's perfect and what we should strive towards doing. Under 0 means you are most likely losing fat which in our busy lives seems to be the exception more than the rule. Over 0…well, welcome to the chub club.

Again, in the book I reference RMR which is truly your "resting" metabolic rate. The reason I use RMR is I am taking into account that you are completely lazy and do nothing but sit on your booty all day! Ok, that's a joke. I know you don't just sit on your booty all day; you must lay down sometimes too! No, I'm just kidding again. I use RMR because I want you to have a base total calories for which you should strive to hit. In no way, shape, or form am I implying that anyone is lazy and does not exercise. I just know that some people, including me, do not have the luxury of exercising every day. So the use of RMR is perfect.

Alright then, let's put the formula into practice, plug-in Elmer's numbers, and see how Mr. Fudge measures up!

8. BACK TO THE FUDGER

Hello Elmer! Let's map out Elmer's scenario and apply it to the formula. This is where everything involving that crazy formula starts to make sense. Plus, this is a great example to help you map yourself to the formula. If you recall, Elmer has a 2,000 calorie RMR per day. A 2,000 calorie RMR divided by 24 hours in day equates to an average of 84 calories burned per hour. That's how I got the "84" value shown below. Remember, this does not include Elmer walking around the office, going to the restroom, climbing stairs, picking his nose, etc. All of those actions contribute to the additional burn of calories. Yes, even nose-picking.

Elmer had 5 caloric intake intervals...ok, he ate 5 times. The decimal number in the below equation, 2.5 for the first part of the equation, that is multiplied times the "84", is number of hours in between the first and second meals. The rest of the numbers map back to the CCI and the RMRFI. Use the formula in the former chapter as a reference if needed. Not that you need it...this is pretty straight forward...well once you go through it a couple of times. Here is how Elmer's day maps to the formula.

$$((400 - 84*2.5)*1.4) + ((300 - 84*2.5)*1.4) + ((700 - 84*3.5)*1.4) + (300 - 84*4.5) + (800 - 84*11) = 758$$

Wow! That's a lot of numbers. Just to help, here is the first set of parenthesis extrapolated. "400" is the calories he consumed for breakfast. "-84*2.5" is the calories he burned over the 2.5 hour period in between meals...remembering that Elmer burns 84 calories per hour. The total is multiplied by "1.4" because the "(400-84*2.5)" was a positive number. Notice that he ate over what he should have 3 out of 5 times...identified by the multiplication of "1.4". So each set of "( )" separated by a plus sign is an interval in which calories were consumed and burned. So five sets of "( )" equations all added together means five meals. Hope that helps.

Applying Elmer's eating scenario to the formula gives Elmer a grand total of...758 calories that could be stored as fat!!!! This could also be stated as 758 calories worth of exercise or fasting in order to get Elmer back to where he was the day before. This is basing Elmer's body being exactly similar to mine. So...do you think his eating scenario is good or bad? Well if he did not do any exercise that day, then it was a fat day! If he exercised, then maybe he got back to zero and no fat was stored, but he would have had to burn almost 800 calories during his exercise...which is quite a bit.

Elmer, just as all of us do, needs to follow this very simple concept, "Eat how you live." Believe it or not, that's the basis for the whole book. What a neat idea...eat according to your energy needs. I touch on this more later, but I just have to go on about this for bit. We tend, and I am completely guilty, to want to eat whatever is in front of us without thinking about what our energy needs are for the day. Our bodies just do not understand what we mentally just pawn off as insignificant. So when we go over our caloric needs based on the formula…we get fat. When we go under based on the formula…we lose fat. It is nature. It is genetic. And it makes total sense. It actually makes perfect sense; we just don't think about it that way. More in the next chapter…I know, I state that a lot…I just want to keep you reading.

Now we stated earlier that Elmer had a 2,000 calorie RMR. He consumed 2,500 calories. That means he was 500 over for the day right? Nope. Since his body is just like mine, and maybe just like yours, and since he ate too much at certain times during the day, more than his body could deal with, he truly went over 758 instead of 500. This is where my formula really comes into play. The meals, for which Elmer went over, caused is body to store the overage as fat calories. The sum of the overages multiplied by 40% is what took the 500 calories daily overage to 758! Ouch!

This is what took me years to figure out. We cannot just count calories over a day and expect to be fine if we get close to our total number (TCSB), but not control what we eat at the intervals. Because if you are like me, then the fat you stored during the day is much harder to take off than if you just ate based on your RMR…based on the formula…based on your energy needs. Quick thought entered my head. My wife would call me sometimes while we were working and would ask me to meet her for lunch. I would sometimes tell her that I could not meet her because I consumed 800 additional calories to be used during my workout at lunch. Her response, "Why would you do something like that?" My response, "Experimenting getting fat!" I won't write down what her response was. The experimenting paid off though…immensely!

This next part is about an experiment I have tried numerous times, and the reason I want to point out this particular experiment is because we all do it. I don't mean we all experiment. I mean we all seem to share this behavior. This experiment proves why counting calories just doesn't cut it. If I eat 1,000 calories worth of food across my meals throughout the day, then eat a 1,200 calorie meal at night...I gain fat...even though I still hit my RMR. That's why knowing your RMR (resting metabolic rate) only gets you partially the way there. That's also why diets that just have you count calories without regards to the formula above just do not work very well. But don't fret. Don't think, "Oh man, I do this so often...I'll never be able to kick this habit!" No. That's the wrong attitude to have...kind of. The reason I state "kind of" is because it is good to realize that something bad is happening. Realizing that something wrong is occurring is the first step needed to right the wrong.

What should you do then on the days you know you go over? Just take a common sense approach. You could either exercise more to help reduce the overage from the day or fast a little more the next day to allow your body to use some of the energy from your fat stores. Aha! We simply do not do that do we? Oh no, the next day is a new day right? Diet starts Monday right? Oh my goodness, how often do we tell ourselves that we'll take care of it "another day" versus acting immediately? Pretty much every day if you are like me...was me...how I used to be...you know what mean. Don't put off dealing with the overage. Putting if off for a couple of days really means putting it off forever. If you consumed too much energy one day, reduce your consumption to compensate the next day. Again, this only applies for non-exercise or light exercise days. If you are preparing for intense exercise such as a triathlon, long run, or long swim for example, follow the advice of your trainer. Because most likely, you are going to need some pretty good overages.

"Hold the phone Dave, are you telling me I have to bring this formula and keep it on my smart phone and enter the data all day?" Yes. Just kidding. NO! Well, yes and no! If I were you, I would do a couple a days to see on average how you do. Don't think about dieting. Don't think about doing "better" than you normally would because you are afraid of what you may find out after the day is over. No. Just do this for a week or so (not during holidays of course) and see how you eat.

You need to record your eating habits for a while so you know what your average caloric intake really is. You may be shocked at what you find. I know I was. You may also surprise yourself...in a good way. You may not be that bad off. If you are really close to your RMR, then you are one step closer to having total control.

Speaking of control...

9. I DREAM OF EATING

Now that you're not completely confused on the formula, but upset because you now realize that, on average, you have a positive TCSB, I'm going to be open and honest because I've been lying to you up till now. Ok, that right there was a lie. I just wanted to make sure you are still paying attention. This chapter is great. So if you think the book is no good, just wait till you read this part. Hold on...did I word that wrong? This chapter KICKS NEURONS BABY! There, that's a little better. This whole chapter, just like the previous one, helped to change my life forever.

Did anyone notice the subtitle of the book? This whole chapter is dedicated to defining and understanding the "6th sense of eating." Let's start with dreams. I know, "What? Dreams? Surely he can't be serious." I am serious, and don't call me...fill in the rest if you can. How can dreams relate to eating? Immensely. Let's explore.

I've had three types of dreams. I've had subconscious, conscious, and lucid dreams. A conscious dream is a dream in which you know who you are, you know the people in your dream, you do not have total control in what is going on, but you have some thought process in what is occurring or what you are doing. This type of dream can be wonderful or a nightmare because everything in it is mostly realistic.

Now lucid dreams are the coolest and most exciting. In my whole life, I've only had three lucid dreams that I can remember, and they are vivid. A lucid dream is a dream in which you actually realize you are dreaming. The drawback, at least for me, is that once I realized I was lucid dreaming, the excitement, or jolt if you will, is so strong that I awoke rather quickly. After waking up from a lucid dream, you spend the next hour trying to go back to sleep thinking you may be able to get back to where you were...not going to happen. As an extra tidbit, I wrote a short story about one of my lucid dreams and added the story to the appendix. Pretty exciting. I think you'll like it.

Now the last one seems to be the most common; a subconscious dream. A subconscious dream is a dream in which you have no idea what you are doing. You mainly have no idea who you are. You have no idea who the people around you are. The whole dream, really, does not relate to you at all consciously, but may relate to something that you read about, have seen happen, etc. A subconscious dream is the dream that when you wake up, you go, "well that was completely stupid." You feel lost and confused after a dream like that. With me, it makes me feel dumb because I think to myself as to why I didn't try something different in the dream. But these dreams are driven from the subconscious part of the brain for which you have relatively little control...hence the word...subconscious.

So now that I described some of the different types of dreams, how do dreams relate to eating? Dreams help define characteristics of the 6th sense of eating. Ok…so we are finally here. WHAT IS THE 6TH SENSE OF EATING? Simply "processing information" before, during, and after caloric consumption intervals (CCI) in a fully comprehensive, conscious manner. What a bunch of mumbo-jumbo. The 6th sense of eating is just thinking about the eating process before, during, and after each meal. Why do I always make the first attempt so complex when defining things? Think about it…we use the 5 senses easily when eating, but the 6th sense seems to be the most difficult.

Now I want you to stop here for one minute and truly ask yourself this question, "Do I consciously think about the eating process when I eat?" It may not be too surprising, but almost every single person's answer is a resounding "No." Don't feel bad though. It's a learning process; trust me, it gets easier. Very few people "actually" think about eating while they eat, and equally as important, think before and after they eat.

Most people, including me not too long ago, treated the whole eating process as a subconscious dream. We are like mindless zombies out there. We are hungry…we get a bunch of food…we eat as much as we can and as fast as we can. Maybe we are talking to someone or worse watching a movie, and never realize what we are doing. Anyone who has ever eaten a meal, and then got in the car or sat on the couch or stood up in dizzy stretch and thought, "Oh my goodness. I feel nauseous. I feel dizzy. I feel like I am about to pop or throw up." YOU ARE GUILTY OF BEING A SUBCONSCIOUS EATER!!! Don't feel too bad after reading my ALL CAPS sentence; you're not alone. I have not met a single person who does not do that at least once on a weekly or monthly basis. That is subconscious eating folks. That's what we DO NOT want to do. So why did we do it? Why do we still do it?

We still do it because we have not realized that eating is a process just like an obstacle course. Your eating process must have a plan of execution to be done correctly. I did one of those mud-style runs recently. You know, the type of run that is 5 kilometers and takes you through 25 different obstacles, some extremely challenging, half of them for which you are buried in a pool of mud! In that type of event, you just don't take off full blast without thinking. Your energy will be spent by third obstacle. You must have a plan of execution, and you must follow that plan. The same goes for eating.

Subconscious eating is what is causing most of the obesity in our great land. I don't listen to politicians about eating; ever notice how most of them are fatter than their constituents? I don't listen or believe when someone tells me that soft drinks and potato chips are the cause of obesity. That's simply not true. You could eat 15 organic avocados a day and become obese, and I love guacamole! Soft drinks and potato chips cannot make you fat…they are inanimate. "We" make ourselves fat by consuming too much of something with too many calories too often. We don't follow the formula…we don't eat how we live.

Don't get me wrong. I know different foods are literally processed differently by the body, and some foods are more nutritious than others. But I'm not here to debate that. I am here to explain why the enormous amount of calories we consume from subconscious eating, basically not using my formula, is why I see fat people.

Why is conscious eating a little better? Answer…our brains are involved…well a little. I know many people who are conscious eaters meaning they still eat way too much, but they do not gorge themselves like mindless zombies. Conscious eating is when you are at a party, for example, and food is abundant, but you sit back and realize that there is no rush to eat and the food supply will not run out. You are in control, somewhat. This is just like the conscious dream. You kind of know what is going on, but you have a very hard time controlling your eating behavior. Now, let me break here for a minute. I'm no drill instructor. I know that sometimes when the food is awesome, you just have to splurge a little. I hate the word "splurge"; you'll see why in a bit. But just because the food supply is endless doesn't mean you have to pretend the space in your stomach is endless too! I was always notorious for walking around at a party and constantly walking by the food buffet. Every time, I would take one or two items from the buffet and eat them even though I knew I was not hungry at all. Argh! Why did I do that? Because my 6th sense was only partially conscious.

Now, here is what we are trying to achieve, the true 6th sense of eating…*LUCID EATING*!!! Lucid eating is a term I created which means to fully comprehend the eating process. Lucid eating is using your brain to comprehend all accompanying aspects before, during, and after all caloric consumption intervals. I know I just quickly touched on subconscious and conscious eating. Here's why. Subconscious eating is of course the no-no. Conscious eating is only using a part of your brain. So lucid eating is the end result or "nirvana" for which we want to be immersed. So let's dive in!

First, lucid eating is simple. Remember who I am. I was able to figure it out based on the results my body went through during various tests over a two year period. Here's something to throw out real quick. One holiday season when I was just beginning to be truly comfortable with my lucid eating, I lost 2 pounds!

How is that for proof that it works wonderfully! I'm not trying to gloat. I was shocked and extremely happy. I just ate what I knew I should. For everyone out there who's never heard of the term lucid, it really just means to fully comprehend and understand. That's why I love it; a short word with a very powerful definition. Truly, lucidity is about having clarity in the topic at hand. But more than that, being lucid is comprehending and understanding possibly complex processes without having to focus on each detail individually.

How about an example of lucidity that does not involve eating? How about driving to work? Seems pretty simple right? How many steps would it take to drive to work? Three or four? Seriously, this is a cool exercise. Truly stop and think about driving to work. This should take you all of ten seconds. Ready? Did your results come out to something like this?

1. Get in the vehicle.
2. Leave my house.
3. Drive to work.
4. Park at work.

Well that's how I drive to work. Notice how simple everything is? That's because we're not actually in the process of driving to work; we are sitting here reading a book and thinking about driving to work. When I drive to work, the following is really what my brain goes through. Quite a bit different, don't you think?

1. Get in the vehicle. But first, walk around the truck and let my eyes look for anything out of the ordinary like dents, broken items, flats, etc. Ensure nothing is behind my truck before I back out. Buckle up. Turn on the truck. Ensure all gauges are reading normal. Listen to the engine for signs of trouble. Make sure I can see out of all of my mirrors. Make sure everything I need at the office is with me so I do

not have to turn around and come back later.

2.   Leave my house.   Back out of the driveway slowly. Be vigilant and ensure the neighbor across the street has not parked the car, again, in the pullout angle of my driveway making it almost impossible sometimes to get out which really irks me. Before entering the street look all the way around for vehicles driving through the neighborhood.

3. Drive to work. Go up to the stop sign. Ensure none of the crazy kids are zooming through the stop sign on their way to school. Check for kids near the road waiting for the bus to ensure they are safe. Head to the main road. Kick in the brain and the "merge into traffic process" to get my big truck out on the road in a safe enough spot. Slowdown in the school zones and ensure no kids are near any kind of school crossings regardless. Watch my speed limit at all times. Be aware of bad parts of the roads and crazy people darting out of their subdivisions like I just did. Take the easy, longer, less traffic way to work.

4.   Park at work. Pull into my parking lot. Look for a place to park that's a ways away from the door just because I hate being lazy and parking right next to the entrance. Ensure I am pulled all the way into the parking space so someone doesn't back into my trailer hitch that I have been meaning to take off for the last 3 years. Make sure I'm straight. Do one final check of the gauges. Turn off the truck. Make sure I grab all of my stuff out of the truck before heading up to the 4th floor, taking the stairs by the way. Before opening my door, ensure no one is around to mug me or rip my door off from pulling into the parking space next to me too fast. Get out of my truck. Close the door. Lock the door while walking away with the remote. Check the truck from a distance to make sure everything looks ok. Go into work.

Any different from the first 1-4 list? Quite a bit

more because the main items (1, 2, 3, & 4) are what we think about at first because it's the simplest. We were not focusing on what really happens, just on the main points. All of the sub-items, detailed in the second 1-4 list, are what our brain actually does. Weird isn't it. You probably do the same thing, but you just don't realize it.

Learning the methodology in which I drive to work may have taken me a long time to initially develop, but I did it. And I don't mean the actual driving part; that's simple. I mean doing all of those checks and activities that happen before, during, and after driving. The same thing applies to lucid eating. It took a long time for me to make all of my eating decisions a second nature task where my brain, like driving, just knows what to do.

While I was learning how to eat, that sounds funny coming from an adult, I literally had to mentally acknowledge each sub-step. Now, it's just part of my natural eating process. I think back to what I used to do. I really just did the simple steps: I want food, I eat food, done. Sound familiar? Don't worry, your brain will eventually work that way too...the lucid way I mean.

Now, I don't want to make this sound like it's nothing and that you'll pick it up right away. That would be lying. The first couple of weeks is going to be difficult I can assure you. Why? Because if you are like I was, you are so used to stuffing your gut at every meal. Not stuffing yourself is going to feel a little strange I promise. You will be full, but you may feel like you need to eat more. This is where lucid eating really takes hold; focus. You will want to stay sitting at that table and finish your plate because it's still there...and there is still food on it. So you will have to realize that you are, in fact, full and are done with your meal and just walk away.

Let's explore this more…shall we?

10. I'LL TAKE A SIDE-OF-LUCIDITY BEFORE THE MEAL

Change is...wait...change "can" be good. Not all changes are pleasant. Let's promote some good changes and review our lucid eating processes by doing something we all love...going out to eat at a nice restaurant! I will not kid you this time, lucid eating at a nice restaurant can be extremely challenging...at first! Our scenario is a nice restaurant, not fast food. "Nice," of course, is subjective. Let's just think of a restaurant where we think we can get a good, balanced meal.

Ok, what is the first thing that pops into our heads when we go out to eat at a restaurant? Well if you're like me, then you think, "Since I never get to go out I am going to splurge...what am I hungry for?" Well? Did I hit the nail on the head or what? I bet 99% of the people reading this book said the same thing!

How about these questions. What am I hungry for? What do I feel like eating? What looks good on the menu? What's the special? What haven't I had in a long time? What are you having? What's good here?

What is this place known for? All of these questions, or some variation, enter our heads. Sounds typical right? Yep, and this is exactly our problem! This is what we think; sadly, this is the extent of our thought process when it comes to eating. We do not think about our caloric intake for the day or if we "fudged" and we are playing catch-up. We do not think about if we are over or under our RMRFI or RMR for the day. I state RMR here because if we are going out to eat, it is most likely at night, and we will not be exercising later that night. We act like wild animals, "ROAR! GRUMBLE! GIVE ME FOOD!" We totally lose the fact that humans have the ability to reason; well, most humans.

Ladies and gentlemen, this is common thought. Don't feel ashamed. And if you just said, "I don't," then you need this book more than anyone else because you should have felt some shame. I know I did. You should be able to realize a problem when you see it...or read it. Not having the ability to reason and choose a meal that best fits "how we live" relates to the same issue when we look in the mirror and do not see ourselves as out of shape. We may be 30, 40, 50 pounds or more overweight, but when we look in the mirror we only have one vantage point; so we tend to not focus too hard. We tend to not comprehend the problem because we do not work hard enough to see it.

Quick thought. Remember algebra? Some of you went "Aahhhh...math!!!" Don't worry, we are not doing more math. In algebra, you know what you start with and you know what the end result is, but getting there is the problem. We have part of the problem "X", the answer is "Z", so we have to figure out "Y". "whY" is the toughest part of the equation.

SPLURGE! SPLURGE!! SPLURGE!! That word sounds fat doesn't it? It almost sounds like a bad body function. We tend to splurge. The problem is we do not know why. What does it mean to "splurge" and why do we associate splurging with overeating? Man…that's deep…and sadly, true. When it comes to food, why do we usually say that we are going to splurge, and what that really means is that we are going to stuff our faces beyond what our bodies can handle. That just doesn't make sense does it?

Where did we go wrong? When did that idea pop into our heads? Let's say we "splurge" every two weeks. But if, for example, we eat a 20 ounce rib-eye, loaded baked potato, steak fries, beer, and cheesecake, we just added over a pound of fat to our body…in one night! You know as well as I do that we do not think about that "wonderful" meal's effects on our body. We will not dedicate more time to exercise to get rid of the fat that we just added. We will not reduce our calories every day for the next week or two. We give ourselves that one vantage point and convince ourselves that it was NOT worth a second thought. The meal above that I just described would average around 1,600 calories or more. For most of us, that's close to our total daily caloric intake. Yikes! I know…enough with the guilt-trip already. But "yikes" just one more time!

So instead of writing more about how horrible our "splurges" can be, what can we do? Come on, I know you cannot be that slow…hello…the chapter name…take a side of lucidity before the meal. That's it. Tap that 6th sense of eating every time you eat, not just when you are going to lunch or eating a meal at home. Use the 6th sense of eating even when we want to "splurge." Why not try the approach of treating the act of going out to eat as the splurge? And not the food. It is very easy to change your mindset so that the act of going out to eat, maybe with your significant other, is the treat. Maybe you had a rough two weeks at work. Maybe the kids have just taken all of your energy out of you for the last two weeks. Maybe you need a little bonding time with your significant other. I'm not trying to be a psychologist here, but make the process of going out to eat the "splurge". Plus, just think about it...do you really want to spend a ton of money just to gain a pound or two that will be very difficult to remove later? Of course not. It seems that our mindset is just not correctly aligned with planets of the food universe.

So here is what I try to do; maybe not every single time, but a majority of the time...that's for sure. Hey, I'm not perfect either! Number 1, always drink water with your evening meal. "B", never look at the menu while waiting for your drinks. Now, you are probably thinking, "What?" That is the oldest trick in the book by the restaurants. They let you salivate over the menu while you are waiting for drinks, and possibly order an appetizer because they know we are "starving". They also let you wait because it gives you more time to smell the aroma in the restaurant. It gives you more time to look at all of the "really tasty" dishes on the menu or on the table next to you. My advice, leave the menus flat on the table. Do not open them at all. Once you get your water, kindly tell the waiter, that you need about 5 more minutes. Hey, the world is not going to end...I mean, I can't promise that, but hopefully not. Drink 4-8 ounces of the glass of water and wait for a minute or two. Enjoy your "splurge" for a minute. Talk about something interesting or whatever. If the approach of drinking plain water on a completely empty stomach just feels weird, then order a very light salad first before ordering anything else. Then after eating the salad, wait a minute or two.

NOW, you may open the menu. What you will find is that you are no longer looking for the largest chicken-fried steak on the menu or the triple-bacon, triple-cheese, cheeseburger either. What you'll find is that you tend to want to eat a little less. Many times, my wife and I will order two small dishes or one larger one and just share the meal. Regardless, when the meal ends, you hopefully only consumed what you needed, and you feel "full" and not stuffed like a piñata.

Now seriously take a minute and try to let that soak in. You can use this same approach any time you eat. Remember the 6th sense…remember to "eat like you live." Remember to lucid eat where you are in control before, during, and after the meal. The reason the paragraphs above are so effective is because a growling stomach does not necessarily mean you are lacking calories…it just means your stomach has no food in it to digest. That's it…right there. That is the first step in lucid eating, understanding what is happening with your body even when those embarrassing wolverines are fighting in your gut; at least, that's what it sounds like. If you estimate you are 600 calories away from breaking even for the day, then try to eat 600 calories or less. What good is 1,200 calories going to do you if you are just going to go home later and crash into a digestive coma? None. Realizing what you NEED is lucid eating.

So before the meal, try to curve your appetite slightly just to stay in control hence the half glass of water or the light salad. Next step, what to do during the meal? Well first is to not snort your food into body. Slow down. Enjoy the company or the scenery or the ambience, etc. Eat slowly and drink water while you eat; it truly helps to aid in digestion. Plus when you drink water with your meal, it actually helps make you feel full faster because water can speed up absorption. Quicker absorption truly curves your appetite. Chew your food more than twice before swallowing. I swear that was my worst problem with eating…still is sometimes. I tend to eat way too fast like someone is going to come steal my plate from me mid-way through the meal!

Continuing on, spice the food. Of course, the process of spicing your food is very subjective, but I'll give you a quick example. The other day I went out to eat after a family event and had a bowl of Cajun seafood gumbo…saliva is starting flow like a Pavlov dog…I love gumbo! I only ordered a small bowl of gumbo. So my 6th sense was working great. Why? Because I was about 300 calories from breakeven. Now I know…I should practice what I preach. But I love almonds, and that day I just ate too many towards the end of work. Don't get me wrong, almonds are good calories, but calories nonetheless. I knew this bowl of gumbo with rice would be about 400 calories. Of course, I had nothing else with the meal except for a glass of water. I was hungry; I had a small Tasmanian devil spinning in my stomach. But regardless, I thought about what I was doing. I knew I should not eat that whole bowl of gumbo. So I took the gumbo, which was already super spicy, and made it even spicier. I added red chili paste and another hot sauce. I love spicy food, so I didn't mind. Well I didn't mind until my lips were on fire. But eating spicy food usually slows you down a bit. Again, it gives you time to think and watch what you are eating, not to mention the fact that you want to savor the taste. Also, spicy food tends to make you drink a little more water further controlling your food intake and aiding in digestion. Sure enough, I left about half the bowl there with most of the meat gone and most of what was left was rice. Success…even when I felt like I was starving beforehand.

So, do you know what I felt like after eating half the bowl of gumbo knowing full well that I was "starving" before the gumbo? Perfectly full; that's what! See it really didn't matter what I ate. My goal was to trickle charge, and I succeeded. Plus, I had a delicious meal. Another good point, remember what I stated earlier about guilty eating…when you walk away from the meal, and you have to loosen the belt or unbutton your pants? That's not the case when lucid eating…obeying and following your 6th sense allows you to leave your pants in the same position as when you started the meal! I left the restaurant happy because not only did I eat some awesome gumbo, I controlled myself. That control lead me to NOT gain one ounce of weight that day. Completely satisfied…with my meal and my mindset.

So up till now I have stated how I act before and during the meal, but earlier I mentioned that lucid eating encapsulates what you do after eating as well. What are we supposed to do after we eat? I mean, we're done right? Wrong. What does a computer's operating system do before it shuts down? The operating system prepares the computer for its next use. It turns off programs and services correctly. Most importantly, it "registers", or saves off, the information it needs in order to start correctly the next time. And that is how we should be. We need to register what we just ate. When it's not our last meal of the day, the registration process helps us understand and remember what we ate so that we can achieve our TCSB more accurately when eating meals later. When it's the last meal of the day, the registration process helps us determine how we should eat or exercise the next day. A positive TCSB means we may need to take in less calories or exercise the next day; a negative or 0 TCSB means we are on track and are lucid eating! So regardless if you ate over what you should or under, you need to register that information.

Here's a simple question…why do we go out to eat? Heck, why do we eat at all? Answer: To bring energy into our bodies. That's the entire answer. Very simple, but true. We eat to energize; that's it. It doesn't matter if you are eating grilled salmon or a stuffed baked potato; we eat for fuel. We are rechargeable batteries...don't ever forget that.

So compared to other animals in the animal kingdom, what happened to humans and when? When did humans forget that they should eat based on their energy needs? Who's to blame? I blame the French with their culinary perfection. Ok, that's a joke...kind of. But the culinary arts are partly to blame. Food has transformed from a necessity to a luxury within most of the modern world.

I truly believe humans' sense of taste has guided us on a path of misunderstanding...a lack of eating lucidity. We tend to focus too much on taste and not on quantity. Ok, read the previous sentence one more time....then one more time. IS THAT TRUE OR WHAT? And don't say, "What." How many times do we go overboard eating bonbons or pastries and say, "Ohhh....that is so scrumptious!" And there we are...instead of stopping at two or three bites, we devour the whole portion sitting in front of us. GUILTY! Not you...me! I used to say that all of the time. Or I would even lie to myself thinking, "Oh I'm still a little bit hungry" which really meant, "I think there is 1.624 cubic inches of space left in my stomach... let's...just... keep...stuffing... in...food!!!!!" I know; I don't have to even write it. I know what you're thinking. And why? Those darn French! Everything tastes so good. So like a mindless animal, we have evolved into a mindset of seeing the food means we need to keep eating the food. Bad human!

So, how do we combat this culinary conundrum? Somewhere in the book I wrote that change "can" be good. Progress does not always move you forward.

Those who fail to embrace history are doomed to repeat it. Ok, truthfully that was more of a political statement than about eating, but still applies. What I mean is we have to revert back to our roots. We truly have to embed in our minds that, yes, food can be wonderfully tasty, but necessity should come first. Eat for energy, eat for life, and always, eat how you live. Even when the food is super-delicious, only eat what you "need".

Here is something very important…have fun with eating. This book is not about doom and gloom, quite the opposite. You should be able to enjoy a wonderful meal. Notice in the book, I never tell you what to eat? I'm not your nutritional guide. Those decisions you will have to make on your own or at the guidance of a qualified counselor. But have fun. Eating can be an enjoyable event, but just use your common 6th sense. If an eating place you frequent is known for their cheesecake, for example, and you know you are going to order a piece of cheesecake, then order a very small meal. Or eat a couple of bites of the cheesecake and take the darn thing home with you. That's one thing that has always irked me with some of my friends. They would say, "Well I ordered this expensive meal…you can make darn sure I am going to finish it!" No common 6th sense whatsoever. Just get a to-go box and take the rest of the meal home…the same goes for the dessert.

Here is something that is going to totally freak you out…ready? It is ok to leave food on your plate! There, I said it. How dare me! Yes, leave it! You already paid for it. It's not like the restaurant is going to take it to the back and give it to someone else; ooh, gross. It's like the fuel tank on your car. How many people have you seen that just keep clicking the filler over and over and over once the thing has shut off because their tank is full? Oh that drives me nuts!

That .04% of one gallon that got into the downpipe of your tank is not going to help your car drive another 100 miles. Same goes with food. When you are full, stop…but enjoy before you stop! And one more thing along these lines. A piece of cake at a party will not ruin your diet. If you are eating so close and counting your calories down to the nearest 10, you are just strange! I promise you eating a piece of cake or a small scoop of ice cream at parties, for which you go once every two months or so, is ok. The same thing goes for a donut EVERY NOW AND THEN! Do not eat donuts all the time, please. Just keep your 6th sense motor running and know your limits. Do not just quit eating the things you like either. Because the more you stop "cold-turkey," the more you will crave them! So if you are craving a donut, and you are on track with your RMR, then eat one. Eat one, not one dozen. I used to be guilty of that too!

I love the last two chapters we just read! Really. The minimal amount of information in these last two chapters have changed my life. It's almost like an awakening…an awakening of my 6th sense! Please make an effort to read these two chapters again and again. I wrote them…and I still go back and read them again because there is so much attainable knowledge in them…and I wanted to make sure I wrote them correctly as well. Oh yeah, sorry to upset you if you are one of the people who always overfills their fuel tank, but stop that if you are one of those people okay? Sheesh!

Ok, let's flip to something totally different; the next chapter!

11. TOO FAT OR NOT TOO FAT, THAT IS THE QUESTION

Am I a size six? Sure, maybe my right buttock! Why do people try to get to a size? Really. What does that mean anyway? I've heard women say, "Well I was a size 6 in high school. I really need to try to get back to that size." Why? Says who? Where is it written that every woman has to be a size 4-6 and every man has to be a...uh...how do men size themselves? Uh...moving on. I know that this topic is off the "energy" path, but I just wanted to include it because of the changes your body may go through while lucid eating. Plus this chapter has a main point that I really want to get across that is extremely important. So let's continue.

One day I opened up some of my wife's women's retail clothing catalogs, you know, the one's with the really unattractive women modeling the clothes. Ok, that may be slight fib. But then I opened another, and then another, and then another for purely scientific purposes. What I noticed is that every woman in these catalogs has almost the exact same body shape. The women in these catalogs average from a size 0 to a size 6, and size 6 was probably just because of the model's height. Don't get me wrong, they are pretty, and airbrushed. Then it hit me.

What are perceived to be "trendy" magazines and catalogs are setting the de facto standard of what women should look like. Now I know there are other factors for the clothing companies. The clothing companies want attractive women, and they want relatively same sized women so that each woman can model just about any of the clothing lines offered by the clothing company. I get it. But it has become the norm that women, in general, are being judged against a very small sampling of women who model in these catalogs. Now before I upset any of the women in the catalogs, I just want to state that there is nothing wrong with the way you look, trust me. Along the same lines, have you seen some of the tabloid pictures of actresses, for example, where they have gained a few pounds? Their larger than expected body sizes become major headlines, but why? If they are happy in life, and are happy with the weight they have because that is their normal weight, then what's the big deal?

Look, I'm not here to point fingers. This is a book; that would be pretty difficult to do. What I'm stating is for an entity, such as a magazine, to push a healthy lifestyle is one thing, but to push a certain type of body, size, shape, or weight is another. Men are held to the same standard, but since women are naturally beautiful creatures, it seems to me they are treated more with more scrutiny than men. So what is the perfect size for a woman? 36-24-36? Size 2? How about a man? 6 foot and 185 pounds? Waist size of 32 with a 48 inch chest? Those sound ideal, but cannot be achieved by everyone can they? Of course not.

So let's get down to brass tacks. No one, and I mean no one likes being, what has been deemed as, overweight or obese. No one. That may sound like I'm being a little harsh, but it's the truth. Not just for perceived beauty reasons, but for health reasons as well. And the flipside is the same too; no one wants to be as skinny as a toothpick. A severe lack of fat can cause numerous problems as well.

So what is the best size? What is the best weight? The answer...the size and weight that works best for you...and for your significant other. Now you are probably thinking about why I would mention "significant other" where the main focus should be ourselves. The main focus is ourselves, but humans are creatures that crave positive feedback, especially from our significant other. We, of course, want to be happy with ourselves, but when our partner is all goo-goo-gaga over our appearance...well...that's just icing on the cake! But you are correct, the first person who has to be happy is you.

Lifestyle. Everyone has a different one. Some people love to exercise, and some do not. Some people have kids, and some do not. I could go on and on. So what is the process to get you to "your" ideal body type and shape based on your lifestyle? Experiment. Nothing is going to be laid out in front of you as a blueprint for what your body type should be. You will have to figure it out. I believe once you apply the formula to yourself and achieve lucid eating, your body type and shape will become pretty close to what it should be. That is what this whole book is based on...getting your mind where it needs to be first. Your body will follow. Utilizing my formula and performing lucid eating will help your body get to where you want it to be. Exercising will just further enhance your physique.

You probably didn't want to hear that did you?

You are probably reading this book and waiting for me to express to you what the ideal height and weight is for the average person or the exact diet plan. WRONG! I mean, I did state that, but it was just to prove a counterpoint. Think about it; scientifically, almost everyone's body works the same, but it's our lifestyle that tends to be one of the main determining factors for your personal ideal body type and shape. You are going to have to ponder your lifestyle and analyze it to see if it is truly what you should be doing, and only you, truly, know if it's right or wrong. You're reading this book for a reason are you not? See, you are already taking the initiative to review and adjust your lifestyle. Document what you do daily, weekly, and/or monthly. Are there any habits in your lifestyle that will have to change in order to have a positive change on your body? That is for you to decide.

One action I have found that does not work is giving lifestyle advice to people. Some of these questions pop into mind. Is it ok to drop hints? How will the hints be received? Is the person susceptible to change if given a roadmap or guidelines? Will this person hate me and start throwing things at me? The last question is the one I always worry about! Ouch! So many times I feel like I need to tell someone that they are living wrong when it comes to health and maybe their children's health. Boy is that a tough topic to initiate. It's like testing an electric fence by touching it to see if it's on or not! So no, I don't like to do that. But I would bet that most people who need lucid eating will not take the initiative to get this book...someone who cares for them will have to prod them...like you!

Also, many people are in denial. They truly take that one vantage point in the mirror and think, "Oh, it's not that bad," when it truly is. For example, I often see severely obese people at the grocery store.

As I stroll by, I tend to peek into the food horror that lies in their basket. The basket is usually filled with about 80% junk food. One time in line, I just mentioned with a smile, "Boy, that's a lot of food you got there." The lady replied, "Yep, the kids have a bottomless pit." I just bit my tongue and smiled. This lady was very obese; I don't think all of those snacks were for her kids. I felt like I just wanted to hug her and tell her that she can do so much better than that. I know, or at least I think I know, that the lady checking out at the grocery store would like to have a much better body shape. We all have potential, we just have to strive to achieve the shape we want.

So, is there a common body shape that everyone can achieve? No. Some people are short, some tall, some have wide shoulders or wide hips, some are hour-glassed, and some are egg shaped. Need I go on? You are what you are…boy that's a genius statement. My point is, your body shape is genetic. Humans cannot be thrown onto a taffy puller and be twisted and pulled into a different shape. We just have to work with what we have. A human puller/shaper would be cool though!

One thing that truly differentiates us no matter what our body shape, is how we store fat. I have known women with little to no fat on their bellies, but have plenty of junk in the trunk! Then I have met women with lean, strong, muscular legs and booty, but have a lot fat all over their upper body. Women tend to have more variations than men it seems. Most men I know, have the one problem…mid-section fat. That's me too. When I gain fat, it appears on my belly right below my chest all the way down to my hips…very annoying!

So after some experimentation and a little goal setting…AND becoming a lucid eater…you too will find that you have a body type and body shape. Since

I didn't do it earlier, let me give you "my" definition of body type and shape in regards to the topic at hand. Body type refers to the literal physical reference such as hour-glassed or bell-bottom. Body shape is how your body outline is formed from fat storage. A better shaped body can give you more detail about your body type. Regardless, it all works together; that's why I always list them both. I just wanted to clarify that when I state body shape, I am really defining a self-subjective point of view about how you look with your "natural" amount of fat.

Your age, your activity level, your muscle mass, your job, your free time, your average hours of sleep, your...well you get the point... are factors that affect your body and the shape you want to be. Here is the word that makes it all happen - sustainable. That word. That one word is where your focus should be when it comes to body type and shape. Your ultimate goal is to get your body to a sustainable level.

This is the extremely important point I mentioned in the first part of this chapter and for what this whole chapter is based. You don't want perfection. Ok, let me rephrase that. You don't want what society deems as perfection. You don't want ripped abs unless they are natural. You don't want shredded thighs and calves unless they are natural. You don't want perfectly toned arms...unless they are natural. Why you may ask? Because they are typically not sustainable. Being extremely lean, on average, requires a severe amount of work to keep that physique. Plus, that would mean your fat levels are probably under 8% which, to me, is borderline unhealthy.

Sustainability. Keep that word in your head. Make that the focus word when thinking about body type and shape. Do not think because at one point in your life you were at a size 4; therefore, you should try to strive to be a size 4 again. People age. People's body changes, especially women after having children. You may not be able to get back to a size 4. As well, you may, but do not go above and beyond what you think you can do. Why? Because sustainability is the key. The name of this chapter states it all. Too fat? Or not too fat? Pick a place in the middle that you like and can naturally lucid eat to sustain that level.

Our lives are based around sustainability. Overall, we do not want to be overworked, and, at the same time, we do not want to be too idle. The same goes for your body. Reach a level that you believe is good for you and one you can sustain easily within your lifestyle, and above all else a body type and shape that makes you happy and proud.

I know people, LOTS OF PEOPLE who get thin, then get fat, then get thin, then get fatter. This happens when we try to trick our body, such as trying crazy diet plans that only work while you are on them. When you follow my formula and achieve lucid eating, you will naturally get where you want to be. The keyword there being "naturally." Now what do I really mean by naturally? Well, there is a pill for everything is there not? They may help, but worse, they may hurt. Even if the label for the pills states "all natural ingredients" doesn't mean your body will react in a "all natural" manner. If you are going to introduce supplements into your diet, do it with guidance and vigilance.

Now, one big trend I am seeing a lot of nowadays are the businesses that offer a "quick" weight loss solution. Now, before you jump on my case and tell me that your best friend's cousin's boyfriend's brother-in-law did that, and it worked wonders, hear me out! Oh yeah, this is a book…read me out! First, why do you want to lose weight fast? Is your 20th class reunion coming up, and you just now realized that you have a lot of fat on your body that you want to remove before seeing these people? Don't try to impress your former classmates that you are not going to see again for another 10 years. After an event like that, people will talk for a week or two; then everyone's lives go back to normal. No one really cares how much weight you have gained or lost but you. So, back to the point of these weight loss solutions. They may work. They may work well, but are they just another crazy type of diet that just happens to be endorsed by 300 doctors which may or may not have decent credentials that qualify them to have some sort of input on what is a great weight loss process for you? That's a long question!

Moreover, how exactly does the weight loss occur? Many of these weight loss "solutions" only truly work if you take their supplements. Is that natural weight loss? And what about afterwards? Let's say you drop the 40 pounds for which you wanted to lose. How long will it stay off? Two months? Six months? You see, the reason many of the plans end up failing is because it did not require a vast amount of diligence to get the weight off. You were maybe monitored by a physician. You possibly had specialists holding your hand all the way through the process. Ok. What happens afterwards when they are no longer there?

If you still do not understand your body's energy needs per day, $E=MEFAT^2$, and you still have not achieved some level of lucid eating, do you really think the weight will stay off permanently? Me neither. Now a little side note. I'm not lumping every facility or business that offers these processes together. I do believe there are legitimate businesses out there that may work. If they help you experiment and find your RMR, for example, and try to help you learn how to lucid eat, then their credibility is increased. But many of these places, sadly, make their money off of their supplements. So I would have to question their legitimacy. If you choose to go that route, perform due diligence and investigate them thoroughly. I truly believe if you use 1/100th of your brain power and achieve lucid eating on your own, you will be able to control your body's shape and weight to your liking based on "your" choices based on "your" lifestyle!

You see, if you can use my methodology to lose weight/fat by using your own common sense to develop your 6th sense, then you are not getting a quick fix. By achieving lucid eating, you are actually changing your behavior which is where the problem lies anyway. Your fat was not the problem...how you treated food was/is your problem. Plus think about it. If you take control and get your body back to a sustainable level that you enjoy and can live with for the rest of your life...uh...YOU DID THAT! Not someone else. Your attitude will be better. Your outlook on life will be better. You'll become a role model. All because you made the decisions which resulted in positive actions that are of your control and not some pill. What is better? To be given a fish or to be taught how to fish? Another positive...when you achieve lucid eating and get your body back to your defined sustainable level, you will not be worried about how you will keep the weight off once the "plan" is over. Lucid eating is not a plan that ends; lucid eating is a process that stays with you for life.

I've heard people ask, "How do you achieve sustainability?" You know, that's a really good question. Answer: Do the opposite of our federal government! Ok, all seriousness aside. What are some good tests for sustainability? How do we know if we are sustaining? You could use a tape measure or fat calipers and record your measurements. There's always the weight scales too. I typically fluctuate 3-5 pounds per day depending on how much fluid I drink, salt intake, etc. So I just ensure that I am within my range daily. How about some everyday non-scientific tests to measure sustainability? That can be easy, more realistic, and less of a hassle because truthfully, most people do not care about how many millimeters of fat they have on their love handles. Buy a pair of jeans that you know you "should" be able to wear comfortably. Or how about the pair that used to fit a couple of years ago that have been on your closet shelf collecting dust?

After you start using my formula and achieve a good level of lucid eating, use the jean test. Try them on every week. Do they fit well? Too tight? Too loose? Since I don't believe in trapping ourselves to a particular size, determine sustainability by how well your current clothes fit. Stop wearing the baggy shirts, and get something more form fitting as a continued test. Then you can see where you may be lacking or where you are excelling. You don't have to wear the form fitting clothes out in public if you are not ready yet. Just use them as benchmarks. Use multiple mirrors and not the one vantage point, remember? Review yourself with clothes on and NOT off. The reason I say to review yourself with clothes on is because our skin tends to be a little more fluid or forgiving in the mirror where clothes reveal quite a bit more. For men, form fitting shirts in multiple mirrors usually does the trick. We can see the "party ball" pretty easily. For women, tighter clothing or bathing suits work just as well. Remember, you are not trying to be that 20 year old size 0 model in the clothing catalog or the guy from the latest fitness magazine…you are trying to be a happier, healthier you.

What really shocked me one day, and made me proud of myself, and made me realize that lucid eating truly works, and this is a run-on sentence, is when I looked in the mirror after getting dressed and thought

I looked nerdy. Sounds funny I know, but what made me look nerdy was the fact that my belt buckle post was in the next to the last notch...on the inside! So I had this long band of excess leather from the belt hanging out of my jeans loop! I laughed, and smiled, and thought, "OOOOOOHHHHH YEEAAAAHHHH!!!!" Time for a new belt...and a smaller belt at that! I laughed too because I remember the hand-me-down belts I would occasionally get from my older brother which would fit me the exact same way! But you see, it's the little things you notice that make a huge difference in your attitude and your life. My formula worked wonders for me. Just one more notch in my belt...literally!

So let's see how our belt can get even smaller!

12. COUCH POTATO, COUCH POTATO, WHO IS THE COUCH POTATO

Does the title of this chapter make you want to grab a bag of chips? Actually, quite the opposite. This chapter is about getting the "potato" off the couch. Yes, it is here...the dreaded chapter about exercise!!! If you thought the other chapters jumped around quite a bit, you haven't read anything yet; this one really jumps...get it? Jumps...exercise. Ok, I agree, that was very poor joke. But don't worry. Remember the introduction? I am not going to give you exercise routines; just having a quick, fun discussion. I do mean "fun" because I'm going to jab at some people pretty hard, so don't get upset if you are one of these people. I apologize ahead of time.

During the last couple of championship games for any sport, do you know what I noticed about all of the "crazy" fans? Almost all of them are all fat! That sounds mean, but I thought it was hilarious. I mean, you have guys who know everything about everything about every player in the sport, and they are like 100 pounds overweight. I want to scream, "Quit watching the sport and get into the game…literally!!!!" There it is. Our first topic; entertainment.

Has it always been like this? Since when has sports become the dominant form of entertainment? I guess since the Greek Coliseum; so, it's been awhile. I thought sports was something we participated in to prove ourselves to ourselves and make our family and country proud. Is that not the case anymore? Why do all men and some women judge themselves among their peers by how much sports knowledge they have? Take this excerpt between two guys at the water cooler:

<u>Brod Chestly:</u> "What's up? Did you catch the game last night?"

<u>Maximus Johnson:</u> "Are you kidding? Sure I had a late night at work where I do nothing, but I DVR'd it baby! I was headed to the gym for a workout, but stopped off at BadBoy Burger instead. You won't believe this, but I did it again…I finished the 1-pounder with 6 slices of cheese and 3 kinds of spicy mustard and ten strips of bacon! I think I had about 20 new hairs on my chest sprout up last night while I was sleeping! I mean only a 'man' can eat that kind of meal!"

<u>Brod Chestly:</u> "You are the big man, no doubt about that."

<u>Maximus Johnson:</u> "I wouldn't say I'm big. I think 345 is a little above average. Look how muscular my jaw is?"

<u>Brod Chestly:</u> "Maxi, did you see the play where Jimbo Jackmaster did a 360 around the weasel, broke 4 tackles, super high-stepped, and after scoring dunked the pig skin over the h-bar?"

<u>Maximus Johnson:</u> "Oh yeah! I totally watched that play like 50 times. Jimbo is on my fantasy football

league. I wish I could add the 50 touchdowns to my fantasy team! Ho, ho, ho. That would be radical."

<u>Brod Chestly</u>: "It sure would. Hey, isn't Jimbo the record holder for most single carries which resulted in a score from within the defender's 40 yard line before 4th down in the 3rd quarter immediately after a punt return?"

<u>Maximus Johnson</u>: "You darn right. And while he was at Manly State University, he held the all-time rushing record for a junior on a partial scholarship while being a teacher's aid and driving the school bus as an extra job to make ends meet...who was also taking 6 classes that semester! And in his sophomore year, remember, his mother had that bad car accident, and he still never missed a practice!"

<u>Brod Chestly</u>: "I remember that like it was yesterday. I got tickets for next week's game. You up for it?"

<u>Maximus Johnson</u>: "I wouldn't miss it. You know who's coming to town right?"

<u>Brod Chestly</u>: "Oh yeah! Dirk Dugan who leads in all-time QB sacks for a sophomore at away games played before 10pm on turf!"

Ok. That story was fiction...in case you couldn't tell by the guys' names. But doesn't it ring true with many men who just happen to be overweight? They cannot walk for 30-40 minutes a night or concentrate on what they eat, but they know every statistic for every major player on every major team. That's why I can safely say that "sports entertainment" is a very large contributor to the "fat" movement even though it seems like an oxymoron. Seriously, go to your local chicken wing hangout style sports restaurant, bar, thingy. What are they doing? Watching sports, high-fiving, screaming "oh man" 500 times, eating greasy fries and greasy chicken wings, and drinking beer. Tell me I'm wrong! But it's not just sports entertainment, it's the entertainment industry in general.

It seems we have fifty drama or comedy shows and an uncountable number of "reality" shows that have taken over. When did this happen? I recall, when I was younger, reading "The Plug-In Drug" by Marie Winn. At first glance, I thought the story was way over the top. Far too "conspiracy" for me. The story was basically about the destruction of society because of television and television programming and the effects it has on developing children. That's crazy right? That could never happen could it? I mean, please, kids watching TV all of the time, playing video games, movie after movie after movie...what harm could that do? Plenty! Read her findings; the findings will frighten you to death. After reading that, you will ban your children from watching most of what is on TV. So let's jump back to topic.

How does this relate to us now? Immensely, and for this book we are going to discuss the "fat" problem associated with entertainment; more importantly, how entertainment stops us from exercising. I've heard even some of my friends say, "But that's how I unwind...that's my 'me' quality time." Seriously? Sitting on your rear, most likely eating a "quick meal", and watching some horribly unrealistic, usually spoiled-brat-laden show, is the way you unwind? That's a crockpot of lazy stew, and they know it. So let's get this out in the open and state the obvious. On average, "exercise challenged" (lazy) people tend to overeat. That may sound a little mean, but it's true. Why? I guess there are numerous reasons. I think being lazy leads to overeating which leads to weight gain which leads to lack of energy which leads to being lazy...and there we are. So how can we solve this problem?

Well, I'm NOT about to tell you what exercises to

do (remember the Fatroduction). I'm NOT about to tell you how long you should exercise when you do exercise. And I'm NOT about to tell you how often you should exercise. Why? Why won't I give you any exercise tips? Because exercise is NOT mandatory for fat loss!

You read me! That's right. I wrote it. Before you go nuts and yell at the book again saying that you thought this chapter was about getting the "couch potatoes" off the couch, which you are correct, let me give you my opinion first. I have truly found that exercising, in general, is for two purposes: one, to keep you physically fit so you can do the things you love to do or need to do in the case of your career, and two, to keep you moving. Now pause...........and think. Why do we exercise for what we do? To build strength and endurance right? I believe you should only build strength for the processes that you do that require strength. You should build endurance for the processes that you do that require endurance.

Many, and boy do I mean "many," people have told me that they exercise and exercise and exercise and exercise and cannot drop the weight. My head screams, "WHAT ARE YOU THINKING?!?!?" I'm going to state this as plain as I can. You "SHOULD NOT" use exercise as your key weight and fat loss process! Don't do it. Don't fall into that trap. If you do not use your 6th sense and lucid eating to control your body's fat content, you will never win the David versus Goliath battle of exercise versus fat. Exercise is for the two general purposes for which I just mentioned. That's it. Now exercise can be used to assist you when you start lucid eating to help you get the fat off a little quicker, but be careful. You should understand the formula and know all of your formula parameters, like your RMR, first. Once you know and can control your formula via lucid eating, then exercise is a great benefit. But when exercising, exercise caution as well. Think about "why" you are exercising.

Let me give you an example of a person who was just not using common sense a few years back, and now he's writing a book. That's right, me! I got on this weight lifting kick. I thought that lifting weights is what makes you healthy and keeps you in good shape. Well, of course, I got stronger and stronger. Before I knew it, I was lifting very heavy. I thought I was tough. I was looking good. I could leg press over 1,000 pounds and bench over 350 pounds. I thought I was all that. But I didn't realize what I was doing. I didn't realize what the outcome would be.

My common sense was being overridden by the big muscles I saw in the mirror. Now, when I look back, I think about why I was lifting. What was I going to do with all of that strength? Exactly...nothing. I was building mass for no reason. It wasn't going to help me in my job. It wasn't going to help me in my extracurricular activities. But yet, I still lifted heavy. Basically, I was exercising for the wrong reasons. Then my world took a sharp turn...for the bad.

All that muscle, all that working out with too much weight combined with a couple of congenital issues and kaboom! Everything went sour. Too much muscle in the wrong places lead to two severely herniated discs in my lower back. The process of lifting all of that weight created a very strong upper back and neck which ended up pulling my head down towards my back causing two neck vertebras to get so compressed that they started to fuse which pinches nerves and cause severe pain. How do you like that? Or rather, how did I like that? All of that working out....all of that hard work...just to realize I was stupid. Well not stupid...ignorant. I didn't know, or chose to ignore, what would happen until it was too late. I should have been exercising to keep me in shape, and that's it.

So.........back to exercising general purpose #1. I now exercise to keep me physically fit so that I can do the things I want to do. I'm still trying to get that bulk off. I thought it was easy to lose muscle...not so much. I do some triathlons now. I play tennis. I run. I walk. I swim. I drink beer...wait, how did that get in there? None of my exercises now involve heavy weight lifting...well unless it's a really heavy beer. And you know what? I have a lower fat percentage now than ever before. Because lucid eating takes care of me. My exercise is for general purposes only now. Sadly, I usually only exercise 1-3 times a week. But my fat percentage stays low because I don't exercise for fat loss. I control it via lucid eating.

So why did I state that exercise general purpose #2 is to keep you moving? The old scientific adage, "a body in motion tends to stay in motion." #2 is the main thing I try to offer people. Exercising to keep the body in motion is one of the key points we as humans have to remember; you have to get that potato off the couch. I truly believe that it is not all about what exercise you do, but rather the fact that you are exercising...within reason. Just be careful. I know exactly what "not" to do now. Trial and error. I try to tell people to do moderate exercises or exercises that help them get stronger in what they like to do. Again, if you do not have exercises that you enjoy, you will have to experiment. Try all kinds of exercises; you'd be surprised at what you may like.

Now I'm going to interject here and state that I believe exercise is extremely beneficial to the body from a physical point of view. I'm stating this because the last couple of paragraphs seems like I'm almost stating not to exercise too often. That is not my intention. Exercise keeps your joints strong and moving freely. Exercise's cardiovascular benefits are extremely important, and keeps blood flowing to all of your body parts, especially your brain. Proper exercise helps with posture, injury recovery, and many other physical properties as well as keeping your heart in shape, which is one muscle we tend to ignore. I didn't want you to think that I am stating to not exercise. Exactly the opposite. I'm just stating that you have to find the exercises that you like, and, more importantly, do not exercise strictly for fat loss. By exercising for fat loss, you will never truly understand how your body is burning calories naturally. What that means is on the days you do not exercise, you will end up overeating, a positive TCSB, because you are not "aware" of what you are doing before, during, and after meals. What I just stated about TCSB is the answer to all of those peoples' problem where they cannot lose weight no matter how much they exercise!

I believe being physically fit is very important in regards to quality of life. I have found, and am living proof, that exercise is not necessary for fat loss which is what I stress in this book, because this book is primarily about reducing fat by controlling energy intake. Keep in mind that moderate low heart rate exercise burns calories from your fat stores. And exercise is very helpful when you have "those days" in which you go over your RMR. So get out there and get moving, but on your terms! Make the focus of exercise to keep you fit, and not for fat loss.

Just as with lucid eating, you will have to lucid exercise as well. Don't say, "Oh great, I have to use my brain again." Yes you do. Remember that drug that you plug into the wall and watch that does nothing for you. Here's one of the principles I try to teach my kids; when you are watching TV, you are being fed. What is required to be fed? If it's food, then nothing; you just sit there with your mouth open. If it's TV, then nothing; you just sit there with your eyes open…and sometimes with your mouth open too. Cut that dumb thing off and get your rear in gear! So yes, you have to use your brain to exercise. You cannot just be fed what to do in regards to exercise. Plus, when someone tells you what to do, it is usually not pleasant. "Give me twenty pushups!"…see. Finding out what works for you is part of the process. If you are able to walk, then walking is perfect exercise. Find out what you are able to do. It's worth it; trust me.

One of the biggest complaints I have been hearing lately is that exercise is not working along with this statement, "Well, I've tried everything…that's just my weight I guess." Come on. You're 20-30 pounds overweight….you know you are 20-30 pounds overweight….you know should not be 20-30 pounds overweight. Uh, if you "know" that is not where you should be, then something is wrong. Most likely your 6th sense is being pummeled by the other five! Do not lie to yourself and start believing that somehow your genes changed in the recent history and you are now genetically engineered to be 20-30 pounds overweight. Most likely the reason is age. You may change genetically…just change your mindset to match those genetic changes!

So you can't get the weight off that you think you should be getting off? Can't get down to the fat percentage that you know you should have? Then go back to the $E=MEFAT^2$ chapter, and then come right back. Because all of the exercise in the world will not help you if you do not use the formula and achieve lucid eating. Again, you "SHOULD NOT" solely use exercise for fat loss. Exercise is for the two general purposes mentioned earlier…and is sometimes used as the "catchup" factor if you think you go over your RMR…which I do on occasion. Hey, nobody is perfect.

Remember, your fat reduction is not a lost cause. I was the same way. I was one of those people who told myself, "Hey, I must naturally just be 225 pounds. No matter what I do, it just doesn't come down. That must be who I am." WRONG! I was just not doing what I was supposed to be doing. I didn't understand my body like I thought I did. The herniated discs proved that even further and are a constant reminder of how "not smart" I was. So don't get frustrated; learn how your body works.

Here is a funny observation about exercise that I want to share. I used to workout at a gym and would see the same four guys almost every day. Two would lift weights all the time and two would run all the time. The two guys who lifted weights had lots of muscle and way too much fat because they did not do enough cardio. The other two guys that ran all of the time had more lean muscle than the other two guys and way too much fat. WAIT….WHAT? The guys who ran had too much fat as well as the guys lifting weights only? Yes. Why is that? Because they did not understand how their body works. The guys with too much muscle didn't understand that the muscle only helps burn a little bit more calories. So they would eat a ton of food and carb up before their workout, but never burn it all off.

So what about the guys who ran all the time and were still fat? Evidently, they did not know how their body works either. I believe that they were running too fast. Did "say again" pop into your head? Yep, I think they were running too fast. I mean, those guys would put me to shame in running. They could easily run at a steady 8.5-9.0 miles per hour. That's crazy…especially if you are trying to burn fat. At that pace, they are burning more sugar than fat.

So what did I do? I talked to the personal trainers who were very lean. I asked them what kind of cardio workout they do. I was expecting a 10 mile uphill run or something extreme like that. Do you know what every single one of them told me? They walk for 45 minutes to an hour every day and constantly sip water as they walk! That's it! Nothing strenuous. I thought they were pulling my leg until I started noticing them on the treadmills just walking and reading or walking and listening to music. They never ran, and the walk was at a steady pace.

What most people do not realize is that your body does not burn fat efficiently during very rigorous exercise, at least not for a very long period of time. The body will deplete fat stores effectively at a low heart rate exercise. For me, the heart rate is around 100-120 beats per minute. The only reason I am going into this much detail about the heart rate is because I didn't know what was good for me for the added benefit of exercise to assist in fat loss when I started either. So now, I mainly walk when I want to burn off some excess energy stored from me…uh…not adhering to my RMR and eating a little too much. Hey, what can I say…I make mistakes…but I also correct them!

I used to see "those" people on the treadmills, you know the ones just barely moving, and thought, "Man they are sooooo wasting their time!" Boy was I wrong. Now I see that those people had their exercise planned perfectly. It was me who had the wrong plan. How about you? You have to learn what works for you. If you are totally lost on this one, I would recommend hiring a legitimate personal trainer for a couple of weeks and tell them up front what you want to accomplish. I state "legitimate" trainer because I don't want you to go and get your friend who has a stack of the latest muscle magazines sitting on his coffee table and trust them with your health. They may be ok at training, but they may do more damage to your health than good. Get someone who trains for a living. But be picky. Ask around. If your goal is lose fat, and all the trainer wants you to do is high impact cardio or heavy weight lifting, then find someone else. They should offer a balanced routine…and that's all I've got to say about that.

Ok, one last topic I wanted to briefly touch on is physical appearance. Again, this book is about fat loss and not so much about anything else. I want health to be the primary concern, but I will concede and state that physical appearance does matter. But truly, doesn't fat loss usually lead to a better appearance? Well, most of the time. You may find that the fat was hiding some parts of your physique that my need some cultivating. So if needed, add a little training to enhance those areas as well. Remember, muscle needs energy for activity. So having a little more muscle can help you burn energy a little more effectively.

Sorry for this chapter being so long, but I was too lazy to break the exercise chapter into smaller parts. That was a joke for all who missed it. After all this "text" of exercise, I'm starting to get hungry.

Let's get cooking.

13. STOP AND SMELL THE HOME COOKED MEAL

Funny how we transcend from getting off our rears to exercise in the couch potato chapter to sitting down and eating in this chapter. All kidding aside, I hope you got some pretty good information out of that chapter. If you are like me, comprehending the information in the previous chapter will make a big difference in how you treat losing fat with/without exercising.

So the last chapter was a little preachy. This chapter is different. It's very preachy. No, not really. I hope you find the ideas and observations of this chapter helpful. I'm going take a figurative "step back" from the whole "energy" concept, kind of, and discuss some topics that are once again common sense, but maybe not common knowledge. These topics still deal with energy, but from around-about point of view. So if you think by now that you are a know-it-all because you made it to the last chapter of the book, you are probably right. But keep reading; you are so close to the finish line!

First idea to convey in this chapter is for you to keep your eating receipts. More importantly, keep your fast food receipts. I'm serious. Keep your fast food receipts, grocery receipts, restaurant receipts, etc. Just throw them in a box. But before you do that, write down what you ate if it's not already on the receipt. Then after about a month, open the box and review what you have. It's a good indication of your lifestyle.

Why do I state to keep the receipts? Because so many times, we lie to ourselves and say that we are just "splurging" again and that we do not eat out or eat "that bad" that often. The reason I state to keep "all" the receipts is because you most likely have good eating habits too. So I don't want you to feel too bad when you look at the receipts. I think you are going to get some great insight into your bad eating habits as well as your good ones. Don't just pat yourself on the back for the good meals; acknowledge that you did well and try to promote that behavior. The wonderful thing is that once you know how to lucid eat, you should never have to repeat this exercise again!

Some of you out there in the realm of "book-reader-dom" think you are just too busy for a home cooked meal. That if you gave me your lifestyle and a list of events of what you do all day, every day that I would have to cut you a break and feel sorry for you. Well, forget it. I'm always busy; so I don't have much sympathy. Now drop and give me 20…more minutes of reading!

I understand that some days may be hectic, but every day? Hmm, I do not think that is truly the case. We used to know some people who told me they eat out every night because they do not have time to cook. They would go out to eat at 6:30 and return around 8:15! I know I'm being a nosey neighbor, but it's a great observation. So no time to cook? Are you kidding me? Talking about a sign of laziness and lack of ethic...to put it softly. They could go out to eat for an hour and 45 minutes, but they could not cook for 45 minutes, eat for 30 minutes, and spend another 30 minutes cleaning up? Isn't that the same time? That's BS; BS meaning "beef stroganoff", what were you thinking?

You can go to any search engine and type in "30 minute meals" and get 5,000,000 hits. So get off your butt and sit down and surf for recipes. I truly believe us choosing to create a hectic lifestyle diminishes family value and work ethic. Notice the word I used, "choosing"? Most of us choose a hectic lifestyle, and are not condemned by one involuntarily. We seem to find so many activities to fill our lives that we forget the little things that are just as important. I'm not pointing fingers because I used to have some of this mentality as well. I just know now what it takes to chunk that mentality.

I cherish every meal we eat at our table. I love to be looking at my beautiful wife and my beautiful children all eating together and sharing our daily stories. When we are at the table, there is no TV, no phones, no electronic devices of any kind; pretty much, no distractions. We "splurge" on each other's company. Our family is so close because we share our lives. We share our good times and bad times in a family only mode. There are no waiters; well, besides me and mommy. There are no noisy kids; well, besides ours. There are no zany people in costumes...well...just kidding. It is the most wonderful part of my day.

Not only does this bring our family closer, but it also shows our children work ethic and rules abidance. You may think your kids or family do not care about a home cooked meal, but I would bet you are wrong. It becomes a part of their life too. When mommy or daddy or both are cooking, the kids see that process as...well...the fact that you care. They may not comprehend everything, but the kids know that mom and dad work hard all day. They know that when you come home and cook for an hour in the kitchen to ensure they are nourished properly that you care. They may not express their feelings all of the time, but they love it. The only exception is when we set the plate full of vegetables down in front of our youngest; then we hear, "I don't like that." You have to take the bad with the good I guess. You may not be a gourmet chef; I know I'm not. But every time you cook, it's meaningful. This behavior will become part of the core ethic in your children to where they will not need this book when they are older. Well, unless they get a little off track.

For the single people or couples with no kids, it is all the same. Do not think because I am just talking about how I feel when I know my kids admire me and my wife for cooking, that I am excluding anyone. There is an amazing benefit from cooking; you learn to appreciate what you do and how you eat. You build self-worth and work ethic because cooking...is work. Plus, if you are on the prowl for a mate, then knowing how to cook is a big turn on! My wife can cook! Very attractive, trust me...her and her cooking!

Why am I harping on cooking? Lucid eating. There's that phrase again. Lucid eating is learned quicker and better when you cook. Think about it. You have to plan a meal. While planning, you usually want to have a varied and colorful plate. That means, on average, you will choose a meat and a variety of vegetables. Whether you are an omnivore, carnivore, or vegetarian, it doesn't really matter. The point is you have to think about what you want on your plate. That is a good first step. Second you will start learning what type of food compliments other types of food.

Too, the overall satisfaction of the accomplishment of cooking your meal builds self-worth.

The most important part of meal planning, though, is the content of nutrients in your food to accommodate your lifestyle. Notice that I did not state that the amount of calories in your food is the most important part; because they are not. Your lucid eating process will control how many calories you eat of whatever meal you make. So make your meals count. If you need more calories for a workout occurring later that day or early the next day, then go that route. If you are over or close to being over your RMR, then prepare a meal that is filling, but low in calories or, again, just eat only what you need. Since you are not getting handed a giant plate full of food, like in a restaurant for which you may have paid dearly, you tend to lucid eat a little easier. So keep that in mind!

Don't just be a boring cook either; cook things that are exciting or new. On that note, change it up. Make your meals different. One meal, include a certain type of food, then the next meal, do not. If there is one thing I am big on, it's food variety. Don't cook the same old stuff over and over…mainly because my wife does most of the cooking! But some kidding aside, cooking the same type of food is boring, and it makes you want to stop cooking. Again, research some neat recipes online, and you will be amazed at what you can do. Anyone can follow a recipe…which means…you can make anything for which you can find a recipe.

Most of all, eat what you like provided you make the best effort to make it healthy, or eat it sparingly if the meal is high in calories. Don't switch your diet to something completely different. REMEMBER THE WHOLE REASON I AM WRITING THIS BOOK…DO NOT DIET…IT DOES NOT WORK FOR THE LONG TERM! I love this next run-on sentence. Dieting is just a short bit of happiness before depression sets in when you realize that you are back to the same weight and fat percentage as you were before the diet because you do not like what you were eating while dieting…or missed what you used to eat while dieting. One more time for good measure, eat how you live!

Wow! My one way discussion with you is really going my way. Simply, I just want you to eat smart. So the idea has to pop in your head, "Well what does the author eat?" Answer …. everything! I kid you not. I love food. I love spicy food. I love meats. I love vegies. I love desserts. I love food…period! When I want pizza, I eat pizza. Now, I will leave most of the bread behind because we all know bread is a fat-fertilizer! I used to eat 3-4 slices of pizza before I achieved lucid eating. Now, 1-2 slices; I just drink more fluids and/or eat a salad. But truly, lucid eating allows me to understand when I am full or approaching full cognitively.

Again, what are we trying to achieve by eating? Energy. We have to remember that! WE EAT FOR ENERGY! If I do not need the calories, then why would I eat a lot of pizza? See, it all works. It's really not about will power. You're thinking, "Yeah right!" Honestly, it's not. If I want chocolate, I eat chocolate. If I want a soda, I drink a soda. If I want some chips, I eat some chips. That sounds like I have no will power right? But it's not about will power, it's about using my formula and comprehending how many calories I am consuming per eating interval. I only drink a small soda, eat chips or chocolate when I know my body can burn the calories before the next eating interval.

Remember what I stated at the beginning of this book…that I won't give you workout routines because I do not know what you like to do for exercise. The same goes here…I will not give you a diet plan, because I do not know what you like to eat! Plain and simple. There is no such thing as a generic/general diet. A dietary plan is, literally, defined per individual, per area, per culture, etc. You already have a diet. A diet is truly just the type of food you eat and the quantity of food you eat on a daily basis. This book does not address the type of food, but more to the point of how much of that food you eat and at what interval.

One major idea I want to promote here is that YOU have to understand if YOUR diet is healthy. Why? Because no one, unless you are a child, is going to guide you on what to eat at every eating interval of every day…with that pyramid chart of the different food groups. Remember that diagram? I still do not know who created that thing. You have to make the right decisions. Don't lie to yourself. Don't pretend. You know what is healthy. You know what a balanced diet is. And yes, only you can balance your diet. Again, lucid eating is a mindset. It's a mindset that does not just involve the amount of calories per eating interval per day, it's also consciously understanding the variety and health factor of the food we put into our body. I know that is one thing I did not touch on very much in the book is food variety, but, again, this book is from an energy point of view.

I get fat! Before anyone screams that I, the author, am lying and that I just have a great metabolism, oh no, no. I wish. Then again, I don't; not anymore. I realized something after I turned 28…I was not 27 any longer! What I really mean is that my body just went into old guy mode early. Before 28, my metabolism was descent. I could overeat and not gain too much fat. After 28, FAAAAAAATTTTTT! And it was even harder passing the 40 year mark. Based on the research I have done, I found that after approximately 28 years of age, most men start having a decrease in testosterone; so I had to adapt.

As we get older, our bodies no longer need a vast amount of calories, depending on our exercise behavior of course. So lucid eating is extremely important as we progress through life. I use the word "progress" because most people correlate getting older to the body getting worse. It doesn't have to be that way! Why do you think I wrote the book? I want to share with you what I learned so that your body stays relatively the same as you age. It works. I am living proof that it works. My fat percentage is lower now than when I was 30. Also remember that your RMR will decrease as you get older. This means you will have to adapt. Lucid eating will take care of that for you because you will consciously be aware of everything you do.

Ooh, I just remembered. Here's real good example of "it's not all about will power." There is a deli that I like close to my office. They have a good deal on a sandwich, small bag of chips, and a drink. The sandwich bread is sooooooo goooooooood. So when I do eat there, I eat the bread for sure. I always get unsweetened tea, so that is never a problem. The sandwich is around 400 calories. Well usually for me, that's about all I can take in according to my RMRFI, and following my formula, for lunch on days when I'm not exercising or light exercising. So what do I do? I save the chips and eat them at 3pm. The chips have another 120 calories. So that would put me over my limit if I ate the sandwich and chips at the same time. So I just spread it out over the rest of the afternoon. Lucid eating. There's no law that states we have to eat our chips as we are eating our sandwich. Well, if you live in New York, you may want to verify that.

See how cool it is. I do not diet. I did eat the chips! I just ate the chips…later. I control my weight and fat content perfectly just by using the formula and lucid eating. And like I stated before, I have fat. I want fat. I don't want to be skinny as a toothpick. I don't want ripped abdominals. Why? It's not natural, or healthy in my perspective. I want a fat percentage that does not negatively affect my body's look or performance and one that I am completely comfortable with so when I review myself, "I" feel like I look good...without kidding myself. And when the wife grabs me by my rib cage and says, "Honey, you look so good," well that is just icing on my cake, like the cake that I always eat at parties because it will definitely not ruin my diet!

One last tidbit before we exit. Recently, a medical organization has declared obesity a disease. Seriously? I, personally, believe that is incorrect. I believe that obesity is a self-induced illness caused by people not using their 6th sense. I truly believe that if people follow the simple concepts I describe in this book and learn how to lucid eat, they would have the ability to control their weight through common sense with little to no effort. Again, that's why I wrote the book...to share everything I learned about the eating process with you!

What do you think? How would you rate what you have read? I'd love to see your reviews (hopefully good ones). I have learned so much about myself over the last couple of years. Like I stated at the beginning of the book, everything in this book is common sense based on uncommon knowledge. The information I present in this book has changed my life forever...for the better. Me eating a meal now, is no different than me driving to work. My brain just "knows" what to do. If you did not have this knowledge before reading the book, I truly hope I was able to present it to you in a fun, meaningful manner, and if you did, then good for you! This was so much fun for me. I tried to keep it short. I hope I was successful. Remember, when you think about eating, use your 6th sense and lucid eat, and train yourself to eat like you live!

So who am I…when it comes to fat reduction? I am a guy that realized Fudge is eating normally. I understand I must charge my body correctly so that I do not have to blame my genes for making me fat. I do dream of eating; so $E=MEFAT^2$ keeps me on the right track and stops me from fudging. I take a side of lucidity with every meal so I never have to look in the mirror and ask if I am too fat or not too fat. I don't like potatoes on my couch, but I love them on my plate…especially when I stop and smell the home cooked meal coming out of my kitchen!

(I truly had no idea of how to get 'Disclaimer' into that paragraph…)

The Beginning!

APPENDIX A. LUCID DREAM

"Right between the Eyes"

It is a beautiful night out. My wife and I are walking through an Asian market place after eating our evening meal. We are casually looking through the little shop windows at all of the China dolls, and fine dinnerware. There is a hint of green light all around us from the fluorescent signs above the shops. After a couple of minutes of just strolling around, holding hands, and cracking jokes like we always do, we decide to head back to our car, then possibly to a bar for a drink.

We walk through a dark alley for which all we hear is the sound of our footsteps and drops of water falling from the balconies of the buildings above. An uneasy feeling begins to settle on our faces. I don't feel too vulnerable since I am packing my XD-45 in my shoulder holster, but the scene is a little eerie even for me. We finally make it back to the side street for which our car is parked in the lot at the end of the street. The street lights are far and between, but are a welcome site.

Puff! Smoke appears from a corridor in our flank. The faint light of the smoldering drag glows as a brutish, dark-haired man inhales forcefully. Three other glows appear shortly after. We begin to hasten our pace when we both view the ambers burst on the ground as all of the cigarettes are discarded in a quick movement. Now we're being followed.

My arm begins to sting from the grip my wife now has from the adrenaline for which fear has released into her bloodstream. Her face poses a blank stare at our car which is only 50 yards from our current position. She stares straight ahead. The sound of eight footsteps gains in volume. I loosen my wife's grip, and slowly reach into my jacket to unsnap my blue steal.

Fear gets the best of my wife, and she begins to make a run for the car which is not but about 25 yards away. I, like a pigeon among others, flee with her. But it's no use. The volume of the footsteps increases. I can feel my heartbeat as if someone is bouncing a medicine ball off of my chest. In one movement I release my wife with a guided hand that forces her to retreat to the opposite side of the car and at the same time, a flash, and a twist…and the scene is set. I now have my 45 cocked and aimed directly at the nose of the first would be assailant who is only 3 feet from the cold steal. The only thing I can hear is the fearful panting of my wife whose eyes are now filled with tears.

"Walk away!" I shouted at the man inches from a lead-induced splitting headache. "I won't say it again." After two seconds, which seemed much longer, he advances……..BOOM!!! I didn't flinch. I didn't falter. I pulled the trigger. The smoke from the 45 was still hanging in the air as my eyes started to pick which target was next. Then my wife slowly stood up covering her ears but still crouching from the thunder of the 45. Out of the corner of my eye and as the smoke dissipated, I saw the man that I shot…perfectly intact.

My wife looked on with a quiver in her lip. I stood there in dismay, but with confidence. The other three men stood still with no expression on their face. As I peered back at my would-be victim, his face was expressionless as well. I holstered my gun. My wife asked me what I was doing in a faint, pleading voice. I muttered something very low under my breath. She wearily inquired as to what I said. I replied louder, "I'm dreaming." She looked at me as though I had lost my senses. I saw the horrified stare in her eyes. I grabbed her hands turning my back to the four men without a care. "I'm dreaming," I said one more time with full confidence. Still hiding from the men, my wife whispered, "How do you know?"

I chuckled because at this point I was already getting excited at the possibilities of what could be done in a lucid dream. I turned and pointed to the man that should now be missing his head, "Look at him. I just shot this guy in the face with a 45, and he is still there like nothing happened. That could only happen in a dream." Her frown of insecurity was evidence of her disbelief. So I helped her get into the car, and we drove away.

About a quarter mile down the road I reassured her, "I know I am dreaming...for sure." She replied sincerely, "But how do you know?" "Look out your window," I said smiling. There, literally, three feet from the car was the unscathed would-be assailant running. She cringed and frantically said, "So what?" I explained, "He is running next to our car...which is going 45 miles per hour. It is impossible for a human to run 45 miles per hour!" At this, she smiled and was finally relaxed; even more so when she watched as the man slowly quit running and simply stood on the side of the road staring at us as we drove away.

We traveled a little ways down the highway when

my wife happily exclaimed, "Well what do we do now." "I'm trying to think of something good; a fun test we could do to make this real exciting," I replied. A dim ceiling slowly filled my view. A ceiling fan sat perfectly still. All I could hear was the sound of a waterfall...which was emitted from my sleep aid device. I was awake! Back to reality slowly everything came, but not as a jolt. I felt calm. Then I shouted in a whisper, "Noooo!" I was excited, but saddened that I awoke without getting to test what could have been something amazing in my dream.

I sat for thirty minutes trying to fall back asleep, but stay closed, my eyes would not. Disappointment and pleasure both filled my mind, for this was definitely the most lucid dream I have ever had, and one I will never forget.

The End.

APPENDIX B. WHAT THE AUTHOR DOES

<u>Fast food.</u> I avoid fast food a majority of the time. Why? Because it seems like everything is coated with grease. I just cannot take that taste. Even when I know I can limit my calories mentally, the grease factor just grosses me out. I feel like I want to scrape my tongue and vomit about an hour after eating most fast food. Also, I'm talking traditional fast food here: burgers, fries, tacos, fried chicken, oriental food, etc. Also, one of the main reasons I try to avoid fast food when I'm hungry is because I tend to want to eat fast which does inhibit the lucid eating processes. Most of us tend to overeat when we eat fast, including me. But hey just like I did today when I ate a little too much, I go an exercise a little more just get rid of that excess.

<u>Caffeine.</u> Caffeine helps me keep my brain clear. I can't drink too much coffee because it makes my stomach ache after a couple of weeks. One thing I have learned is that a little caffeine added daily helps burn more calories. As for how many…I don't know. But the minor amount of testing on myself showed

that caffeine does help. I assume it speeds up the heart and makes me a little jittery. So I guess that extra muscle movement really helps. So far, I have seen no detriment to a little bit of caffeine every day. It helps me wake up and stay clear and alert when driving. I definitely do not use it for workouts. I had a bad cramping episode once using some caffeine drinks while playing in a volleyball tournament...never do that again. It can be a very effective aid as a diuretic, which is the exact opposite of what you want when doing long strenuous exercises.

Chocolate. I love chocolate. I really do, but now I go for the dark chocolate. First, dark chocolate has more nutrients than milk chocolate and second, it has much less sugar on average. It took some time to for my taste buds to get used to the flavor, but now, I can hardly eat milk chocolate because all I taste in milk chocolate is the sugar. I just eat a couple of bites every now and then to satisfy my sweet tooth. I definitely do not cut out chocolate!

Snacks in general. I eat about 6-10 times a day. I really do. I just try to eat small amounts to quiet my stomach. Since I am an omnivore, I eat a mix of everything. To keep my caloric intake in check, I eat different types of jerky for snacks. That can be a little expensive, but I have found that jerky is a great food for snacking. First it's made with very low fat meat, so the calorie intake is very low. Second, it's full of protein. Third, it takes a lot of energy to chew it! So I love it. I let it dry out quite a bit more than normal so it's very difficult to chew. Then I break it into small pieces and snack on that for quite a while. It's great, and it also keeps me from biting my nails. I try to avoid most chips for snacking because they are usually fried and contain quite a bit of calories. Some of the baked ones are ok, but I usually try to avoid them because of the extra calories and little nutritional value.

I eat dried fruits and natural fruits (mentioned below) as well as lots of nuts (also mentioned below). I try to get snacks that are in a lot of pieces or that I can break into a lot of pieces because it seems like I am eating quite a bit, when in reality I am not.

Bread. I now avoid most breads, or at least I try to often eliminate bread from my meals. To me, there is just something wrong with flour. I don't know the scientific formula for it, but I think it's something like flour = fat. Really! The sad thing is I love bread, but I have truly limited the amount of bread I eat. I truly believe bread is engineered in me though. I am of Czech heritage, and we Czechs love our bread! But I avoid bread as much as possible.

Fruit. I eat quite a bit of fruit. I usually have at least two types of fruit a day. They are usually blueberries and oranges. But I eat just about every fruit out there. I think fruits are nature's candy. I try to eat fruit in the morning and mid-day. Here within the last couple of years or so, I have been craving fruit at night. I know that is more calories that we don't need before going to bed, but I truly have seen no weight or fat gain by eating fruit at night. Of course, I don't eat that much either. One thing I have trained myself to do is instead of getting ice cream, I eat frozen blueberries. They are awesome! I'm a berry lover.

Breakfast. My breakfast, on average, is organic peanut or almond butter on a piece of toast with homemade blueberry jam. Cooked jams are so easy to make. I can make two quarts of cooked jam in about 35 minutes. I only use half the sugar of the recipe though. I don't like the jam too sweet. You will have to reduce the amount of water you add if you use less sugar because the pectin uses the sugar for congealing effect. Anyway, the reason I eat that type of breakfast is because it contains a wonderful fruit, organic proteins and good fats, and tastes great. I only use one piece of bread that is toasted so I limit my bread, but still have pleasant, crunchy texture. If I don't eat that, I typically have an egg or two either over-hard or boiled. Eggs are an amazing food. Of course we only buy eggs hatched from cage free roaming chickens because cage free roaming chickens are out eating worms and bugs and everything else that makes the eggs more nutritious. If you ever get a good cage free hen's egg and compare it to the caged hen's egg or grain fed chicken egg, you will see that the yolk is a much deeper shade of yellow and smells bolder than a the caged hen's yolk. I always eat brown eggs. I will have breakfast tacos too. I do eat a donut every now and then, but not often. I truly believe that a protein and a fruit in the morning help you throughout the day.

Big Meals & Leftovers. I try to bring lunch almost every day. I find that the more I can do that, the easier it is to lucid eat because I know exactly what I am getting. Too, I hate wasting money on eating out. I have saved so much money by bringing my lunch to work versus going out to eat. So when we do go out to eat, I always bring the leftovers home. Too, when doing that, it's like I get two meals for one price. Many times when we cook big meals, I try to portion out what's left over into 400-500 calorie plates to bring for lunch the next day. That way, when I sit down for lunch, it is extremely easy to lucid eat because I already know what I have in front of me.

New foods. I eat just about any type of food. One thing I think that helps me lucid eat so easily is that I love to try new foods. What I have noticed over time is that people who tend to eat fast food often do not have a varied diet. They are not adventurous when it comes to food. I will try anything. Now, I may end up not liking what I ate, but I'll try it regardless.

People who do not do that tend to always think that since they do not have any idea of what they want to try, they will just go with "old faithful" and choose fast food. I try to stay away from that trap.

Nuts. I had to write about nuts. Just like berries, I think nuts are one of nature's greatest foods. For one, there are so many types of nuts or what's now classified as nuts. I try to eat almonds most of the time because off the research I have done on almonds. There are so many nutrients in almonds. So when I have to snack, I eat almonds. One thing that is great to help me lucid eat is to have a bag of almonds in my desk. I always have at least two or three types of nuts to eat at my desk. When I get a craving for something to eat, I just eat about 10-20 almonds and some water, and I am good to go.

Any food that is visible. Humans are animals. So we have a tendency to eat food when we see food. I keep my snacks in the pantry. I keep my dark chocolate in the bottom cabinet of my kitchen in a jar. For some reason, and I am guilty as anyone else, we tend to eat something as we are walking by it; as if the food has a tractor beam or something. So when you are done with anything, whether it be lunch, snacks, desserts, whatever, hide it. Lucid eating is easier when we have less temptation.

Eating on Positive TCSB days. On days I go over, what do I do? That's a big one. It really depends. The other day, for example, I ate over my TCSB...not by a lot, but over regardless. And worse, that night after our tennis match, I had a couple of beers. So after the beers, I know I was over my TCSB by approximately 600 calories...ouch! Not good. So the next day I ate the same almond butter and blueberry jam on toast breakfast, but ate yogurt and almonds the rest of the day until dinner. I spaced out my food so that I was never very hungry in between meals. I went under my TCSB by at least 600 calories that day without feeling like I starved myself. That does take a little self-control mixed with a little foresight. I made sure I brought the yogurt and almonds with me that morning so I would not get tempted to do something different around lunch time. The lucid eating takes over after a while I promise you. I automatically know to reduce my calories the next day. Usually drinking a ton of water mixed with very small amounts of food spaced out over the day does the trick for me.

Exercise for Positive TCSB Days. More on the days I go over, but related to exercise. If I go over my caloric range, then I will typically do a run-walk-run type exercise. That type of exercise, where the heart rate goes up, then down, then up again burns ready-to-use calories as well as stored calories. Sometimes, I will get the tennis ball machine and go to the tennis courts and hit balls for an hour or so. That is great exercise. The reason I like a ball machine versus another player sometimes is because I can load 150 balls at a time. Then if I really want to burn the energy off, I will turn on the sweeping mode where the balls are also shot side to side making me run back and forth across the court. After 300 of those, I am spent. I got a good practice in as well as burning about 600 calories or more. If I just ate the calories within 2-3 hours, then I will do a pretty hard run to get rid of those calories followed by a slow walk. If the overage calories were spread out over the day, then a good brisk walk is all I need.

Exercise in General. I do exercise as often as I can provided that I can fit it into my schedule. I play tennis mainly now. I still walk and run. In the summers, I definitely hit the pool. Not the leisure pool though; I mean the 50 meter pool. I love to swim. I would love to have one of those endless pools; you know where the water just flows at a steady pace. I think that would be awesome. I could literally swim any time I wanted. Many times, my wife and I will just go walking through the neighborhood with the kids. The kids can ride their bikes or ride in the wagon. Doesn't really matter. The fact that we are moving is great. I still have my home exercises as well. I have a pull-up bar, push-up handles, rolling wheel for abdominal extensions, exercise ball for just about anything, and a couple of free weights. That way if the weather is not good, I truly have another method of exercise readily available.

Eating Everything. Back to what I said about eating everything. I truly eat everything. That's no fib. As far as "bad" foods go, I eat pizza, chocolate, cookies, lasagna, burgers (homemade)…you name it. I wanted to beat this whole fat issue by not changing what I ate. That was important to me. I just greatly reduce the amount I eat when I do eat those foods. Again, I did not want to drastically change my diet to lose the fat. I knew in my brain there was a method to figure out how to do it. But I truly try to not eat foods with really high fat content. I believe that all of that stuff floating around in my bloodstream is just looking for a place to clog!

Potatoes. I eat potatoes. I love sweet potatoes or mashed potatoes or scalloped potatoes. Potatoes are awesome. I don't believe the hype about potatoes being bad. I made sure I left potatoes in my diet. I just don't eat them fried. Because one thing I know about potatoes is they soak up whatever they are in. My favorite thing to do with potatoes is to get about fifteen of the little two inch red potatoes and boil them. Then I chop of the skins into little pieces. Mix the potatoes, the skins, about a half cup of milk, and almost a stick of organic butter with an electric hand mixer. Throw in some sautéed onions, and that is almost a meal by itself. Now I will admit there are quite a few calories in that dish. For that reason, I have a small portion over the next three or four meals. It's a great side dish for almost any meal.

Television. I pretty much watch no TV at all. I will watch movies here and there, but no weekly shows and no "reality" TV. I believe it is truly sad when we feel the only way we can entertain ourselves is by watching TV. Again, the average two hour per night TV watcher is also the average overweight person. TV should not be how we unwind. If I truly want to unwind, I will go into my room, close the door, lay there in a dark room with my headphones on and listen to Vivaldi. In case you are wondering, Vivaldi is a famous concerto composer from the 1600's. His music is simple, light, and truly beautiful. I love his mandolin pieces. I love all types of music, but when I want to relax I listen to orchestra music. Works every time. Too, I love it when people ask me if I watch this show or that show. Then when I tell them I don't watch the shows, they ask me what I watch. I gladly tell them that I watch no TV because I do not get any benefit from it. I usually get the nod and the agreement because they, too, truly get no benefit from watching TV either, but for some reason they keep on going back to the TV. There are other ways to stay informed about worldly events without watching TV as well. Plus, in my eyes, TV really inhibits me from doing the important things like spending quality time with my family.

Medicines and Drugs. I try to only take medicine when I need it. I believe that too many drugs all circulating through your body cannot be good long term. I know that for headaches, there are just some medicines that work. So when I have a bad headache, I will take something. Too, when I do catch a bug, I will take a nasal decongestant because that usually relieves most of my symptoms. I guess what I'm trying to state is that I don't take a medicine at the first site of any type of ailment. I have back and neck pain, but I do not take pain killers. They don't work for me anyway, and I would be willing to bet they have bad long term affects. I have never done and will never do any illegal drugs. That's everyone's prerogative I know, but I choose to keep my body and mind clean. I fear what long term effects those will have. I choose to stay clean.

Cleansing and Detoxification. I cleanse and detox once a year usually in the spring. Even if I eat, what I believe to be, very healthy food, I still believe there are a vast amount of chemicals that get ingested either by the foods I eat or the air I breathe. Our colon is the most important organ to help control our immunity. I keep it clean. Plus, the detox process helps me purge toxins that may be in my muscles and organs. I think massages are great too for helping to release toxins stored in the muscle tissue. It is rare, but when I do get a massage, I literally drink a gallon of water post the massage and over the next 24 hour period. I flush all of that junk out of my system. I see only benefits and no detriments to keeping my "insides" clean. I believe that internal cleansing is one thing most people just forget about. I think many people are so focused on their outer health, but not their inner health. This topic could be a book all in itself, and I'm sure has been done already. I truly believe that many forms of cancer are caused by toxins all accumulating in one place in the body, then mutating the cells in that area. Of course I cannot control where my body stores toxins or truly if it is able to get rid of the toxins, but I try regardless to keep my insides clean.

Happiness. One of the main things I try to do is stay happy. Of course I get frustrated with things, but for the most part, I take life easy. I have never found an instance where getting all flustered and upset helped anything. I know it's easier said than done, but I try. I choose to only get upset at the things that truly warrant it, and when that anger can be used to help lead me to fix whatever is wrong in the right way. I know some people...many people who seem like they live off of negativity. I mean, I see these people every now and then, and the first thing they tell me is how bad things are going, and how horrible their health or job is. Not me, I try to find something fun to discuss or discuss nothing. Like I always tell my wife, leave work...at work. Leave problems at home...at home. Don't carry burdens with you. I don't. I do believe that stress and unhappiness cause people to be bored which leads to them to look for something to do which leads them to food and overeating! So I try to stay happy and healthy!

<u>Sleep</u>. Sleep is extremely important to me. I literally cannot make it through a day without getting at least 7 hours of sleep. Numerous studies have shown sleep to do a multitude of positive things such as leveling hormones, keeping cortisol at the proper level, maintain mental alertness, lowering irritability, etc. Also, when you sleep, you don't eat; which means, sleep helps burn calories. So I try to always get 7 hours of sleep. The problem I have on average is that I am usually interrupted at least once during sleep. I truly wish I could sleep all night without getting up. I have a habit of being thirsty before I go to bed. I just cannot sleep while thirsty. Of course, I have to get up and go to the restroom about 3am. But, on average, I have found that on days I get better sleep, 7+ hours of sleep, my whole day seems better. I have less headaches, I don't feel like I'm starving, and overall I just feel more at ease.

APPENDIX C. FEED ME

I appreciate all feedback regarding the book. I would like to hear from you whether the comments are good or bad. Even if you have a general question about any part of the book, please let me know. This was truly a great journey which led to an even greater discovery. Thanks for reading!

Email: iseefatpeople@yahoo.com

ABOUT THE AUTHOR

I, David Hrncir, being of sound body and mostly sound mind, am a software architect/engineer by trade. More importantly, I am a blessed father of four beautiful children, husband to a loving, beautiful wife, son of two great parents, and a brother, cousin, uncle, brother-in-law, nephew, grandson, and hopefully friend. I love a challenge. The research and experiments I went through for this book were definitely challenging. I'm glad I'm stubborn because I wanted to throw in the towel a couple of times. But I had to figure out this fat phenomenon…and I did. I truly believe developing the 6th sense of eating will help everyone in any age bracket. I am living proof that lucid eating is the simplest form of weight control there is. On a side note, I love to write fantasy-fiction books with a positive twist. So look for those soon.